The White Life

by

Michael Stein

THE PERMANENT PRESS
SAG HARBOR, NY 11963

Library of Congress Cataloging-in-Publication Data

Stein, Michael
    The White Life/ by Michael Stein
      p. cm.
    ISBN 1-57962-025-6
    I. Title.
    PS3569.T3726 W48 1999
    813'.54--dc21   98-34210
                                               CIP

THE PERMANENT PRESS
4170 Noyac Road
Sag Harbor, NY 11963

"Everything is as it should be, nothing
will ever change, nobody will ever die."
—V. Nabokov, *Speak, Memory*

"And again, when I tried to sing of pain,
it turned to love."
—F. Schubert, *Journals, 1822*

For Tobias and Alexander

Acknowledgements

I am grateful to Anne Bernays, Justin Kaplan, Carol Landau and Anna Rosenblum for their necessary advice on earlier versions of this manuscript. Hester's clear thinking and red pen improved every page. Her love and patience astound me.

PART ONE

TODAY, FRIDAY JUNE 5, I am going to meet the man who killed my father. This afternoon I will drive three hours to the town I grew up in and where he still lives. I am going alone, though in many ways I would like to have my family along for the calming effect they have on me; I expect that my reaction to seeing the man will be anything but calm.

He has filled my imagination for years. I have thought of him too many times, at work, when I attended the 1987 NBA playoffs, while watching our cat rip the yellow feathers from a finch he caught last summer, his wide jaws shaking with pleasure, more than once with cotton jammed into my mouth at the dentist's office, when speaking with my uncles at the annual oppressive family occasion. When I've thought of the man I haven't wondered about his emotional well-being or whether he's a good Christian, a hard worker, a devoted family man. I couldn't care less. Yet I've always had an imagined intimacy with him.

For two decades my mother has sent me pieces of my father: a photograph of the two of them at a sepia swimming pool; his army identification card and tin, braille-punched dog-tags; a small oil painting of him at thirty-five-years old in a heavy gold frame, which makes me wonder why he had a portrait of himself done at that age, what he was thinking. These packages arrive without warning and I am glad they come sporadically, rather than all at once, because the surprise is almost always a nice one. Just before she moved into a tiny apartment two years ago, my mother mailed me a copy of my father's death certificate and autopsy findings that she found while cleaning her files. I read through the six pages quickly, mute with the rage that had always been part of my memory of my father's last night. On the bottom of the last page was the name of the man who had killed my father: Gresser. I recognized it immediately, although if you had asked me what it was before I would not have been able to tell you. I put my father's autopsy report in my drawer with no plan to look at it again.

It was only after the events of the last four days, that I took the envelope out this morning (digging under the paper clips and postage stamps and checkbooks) to review the report. Where my name and address were, I saw my mother's distinctive cursive script which for the past two years had only arrived on thin letters, a birthday check for my children, an itinerary for an upcoming trip. The envelope bulged. The pages inside were slippery old mimeographs; the type looked like antique Smith Corona. My mother had included no note of her own.

I remember what my wife said the day I first opened the letter and showed her the contents. I believe she was as stunned as I was. She said, "Leave it to your mother to unload something like that on you without even a word." But I remember I didn't feel my mother was "unloading" anything. In fact, I thought it should have been mine all along, and I wasn't sure what my mother could have written with this enclosure that would have been appropriate, so I said, simply, "Pretty strange, huh?"

After I read through the report, slowly, more carefully this time, I found myself calling a telephone operator in New Jersey to get Gresser's number. I assumed he would be where he lived twenty years before. His work was there, his family was there, and if he was alive, I knew that he would be there. It was impossible to imagine anything else. It turned out that I was right—his number was easy enough to find—and presumably he had not died, although he was sure to be a man in his late seventies by now. Yet when I finally had the number written on my pink sticky pad next to the area code that I had known well from my childhood (I remembered my old New Jersey number surprisingly easily), I was not sure exactly what I was doing with it.

I have always thought of Gresser as my father's killer. I know this is leftover from my childhood, and childish. Killer is a big word and I do not mean to imply that Gresser shot my father, or stabbed or strangled him. After all, I am not going to a penitentiary to see him but to his suburban house which probably has an eagle door knocker and a rubberized black welcome mat. When I say he killed my father what I mean is this: not enough was done.

I'm sure he doesn't think of himself as a killer, but rationalizes, as nearly all doctors do, that what happened was simply beyond even the best effort of his profession. Gresser had seen many patients before my father ever went to him and saw thousands more in his career, but I had no doubt that he would recall my father's name when I said it to him on the phone. Some patients you don't forget.

I know this; I am a doctor too.

•

White is the color people think of when they think of doctors and hospitals, but to me it is also the color of old age, of japonicas, of everything that is empty, of ice and robes. A white stone among the Romans marked a joyful day; offering a white belt was the deepest pledge of honor among the Iroquois, and the white dog was sacred. In the vision of St. John, a white robe is given to the redeemed. White is an imperial color, one of royal preeminence. White is the color of lilies, of pearl earrings left on a bedside stand, of albumin, incandescence, fury, of well-intentioned lies and the leukocyte, it is the kind of magic practiced to counter evil and the antagonist of black infections.

Zeus was a white bull. Interrogation rooms are always white, as are exam rooms. Tuberculosis was the white plague. Angels, ghosts and the power of sorcery all glow white. What could be more ghostly than a hospital, a world without plants and bedspreads and paintings? White-outs occur when heavy clouds hang over fallen snow so that light from above equals the light reflected; there are no shadows. The first girl I ever kissed had white threads fraying from a hole in the knee of her jeans through which my finger touched her skin.

White was the color of the albino whale. Melville wrote, "There yet lurks an elusive something in the innermost idea of this hue, which strikes more panic to the soul than redness which affrights in blood." Ghosts, our kings of terror, are white and exert over us some sorcery, but Melville feared the white phantom albatross: "through its strange eyes, methought I peeped into secrets which took hold of God."

When I was a child, my father told me that a white falling star meant someone was dying.

The painters of hospital corridors obviously believe the scientists who claim that colors are subtle deceits, not inherent in substances but laid in from without. As I walk the hospital halls I often remember that other line from Melville, that white "by its indefiniteness . . . stabs us from behind with the thought of annihilation." The White Life, I call my work.

The laundry room is the whitest place in the hospital. It is a single room inside a beautiful Victorian brick building with stained glass windows. I pass it every morning on the way to the wards.

Inside, large, white baskets on wheels are piled with sheets and blankets and towels. SOILED LINEN ONLY or CLEAN LINEN ONLY are stenciled on their sides. Hanging from the ceiling like great white carcasses are bundles on pulleys. Everywhere are industrial-size containers of softener and whitener to get rid of dried blood on stiff pillowcases. If you squeeze in, you can see the washers. They are like jet engines, turbines turning hundreds of pounds of wet cloth. They make the sounds of hearts. I can feel a great stain being swallowed here; the place is primitive, has fallen far behind medicine.

A single line of long filament bulbs lights the room and the smell is hot and wet like earth. The pipes that bring and take water are dusty near the ceiling. The floor is a mess of ripped white sheets and empty rubber gloves.

Wash, iron, rewash. Day after day. An endless preparation for the new citizens who never stop arriving.

The nights when I get home late from the hospital, my wife is awake. After a decade with me, she is available at my odd hours and she is charitable. She has her own night accent and the heat of an oven under our comforter. Where she's turned gray, it's only more interesting. If I quit my job, I would spend all my time with her.

When she asks about my day, I tell her what I've seen in the hospital using the gorgeous assembly of names and facts we call medicine. I tell her what I've been thinking, and the people I've met and how they want meaningful moments with me. I tell her about the little tactics of deception the visitors of the sick and I use, and how what we are all after, all we want, is to affect the sick lover-brother-friend-patient physically. That's all we want. Families do it through love, and I do it through doctoring.

While I'm with patients, I'm interested in medical facts, and poise. I try to speak with the rhythm of a running boat. What I tell them is often painfully imprecise, when all I mean to do is give them confidence. But in their gowns they're dressed for ruin. *Between* my visits, in the moments of pause among the terribly busy and the hectic, when I'm thinking of patients, I'm thinking about love.

I do not mean love in a sentimental way, or in the sense of the drastic, nasty doctor falling in love with the patient who later reports him to the medical board—driven by love herself, and her inability to separate him finally from his wife—although there is certainly that kind of love in my place of work. I mean companionship, respect, affection, attention, attachment, possession. Some patients have love affairs with their illness because illness has an obligatory grandeur, my friend Anatole used to say. Some patients feel the life of love they've missed when they are finally alone in the hospital. I use 'love' here in the way the Greek language uses fifty different words for love's distinctions (father-son, brotherly, between spouses, of God, of art, narcissistic). The English options are more limited, all meanings packed into our one inadequate syllable.

When I think about love, I mean passion. In the hospital, with death closing in, left in the power of an enemy, patients often feel most fully alive. And so do I as I match their intensity on the way towards life or death. They are passionate in their conflicts and their pleasures, and I am not only a witness but a participant. The very sickest make me fearful for them; at the same time, excitement runs through me, a preoccupation with every minute of their suffering. At the end of a hospital stay I know their intimate business—I have seen them vomit and bleed and piss and fight—things I previously knew only about my wife and kids, people I love.

Illness has lodged itself in the American Imagination as a metaphor for the ultimate experience. And illness has some deep and often odd connections with the hospital setting and the idea of love. "You'll get over it," people say soon after an affair has ended; the same expression is used when one is sick. I once knew a woman who would not make love in bed—she preferred rugs and benches, tiles and grass. Beds are for hospitals, she said. Hospitals used to be built on the tops of hills so as to be separate from the world, a sense of isolation that love shares. Doctors and patients are as irreversibly intertwined as lovers: they can destroy each other, and a complex ecology of domination and subjugation happens every day inside these buildings on the tops of hills. The French call the marriage of doctor and patient *un couple malade.*

I worked for a while in a hospital called Charity. In the Emergency Room, I would count the ambulances and think of the name printed on the patients' johnnies. *Charity*: tender-hearted, kindly, loving. As a doctor, my job is to love them, I told myself: in other words to make them less anxious about both the unknown and the obvious, to overlook their weakness and inability to show gratitude. Love made me useful.

As a young doctor I was not good at love. Like most young men, I found it troublesome and I did not know what to do with it at work or outside. Only when I came to recognize what I was seeing each day at the hospital—sometimes not easily visible amidst the dark arguments and bitter accommodations, the razor-wire defenses, the deteriorations and attritions that the domestic life carries along when

12

it moves into the hospital—did I discover a talent for love. And it took more years until I realized how the loves in my private life were related to what I was witnessing in my medical life. It was not what I was expecting.

Doctoring is the only serious work I know of where the work and the reward come at exactly the same moment. And it is this connection that brings me pleasure. Any doctor who thinks for a minute can tell you about the many ways that love enters their days. I love my patients because they need me. I love them because they want me to save them and because I can't.

As a witness of love (and how it changes), I have become aware of the many things I love about The White Life: the objects in my place of work, the mood of the halls, the rituals, the mail I receive, the memories some patients evoke, the students I teach, and the secrets I hear, the sense of being in two places at once—among the known and the strange. I wait for revelations but it is difficult to overstate the stretches of tedium. My work is like a car ride through a seaside town, checking out all the convenience stores and clamshacks and bait shops while waiting for the tidal wave. I work in a very strange (and sometimes familiar) white land.

It was only this morning—after a sleepless night reconstructing and writing down everything I can remember of this week and how my patient George Dittus has, since Monday, permanently changed my view of The White Life, which has perhaps (if it's not already too late) affected my way of doing things—that I re-read my father's autopsy report and called Gresser.

I came to The White Life because of my father, although I didn't know it until years later. Illness held a special place for me because he died when I was thirteen. Love saves people, and so do doctors, and when I think of saving I think of my father and I think of medicine.

As I eat my turkey sandwich and drink an iced tea before getting into the car this Friday afternoon, I think maybe I can just begin to understand what I want from

13

Gresser, although I am not certain, of course, what I will say to him once I get there. I want to know the events of my father's last night. Only Gresser knows the details, and I want Gresser to have a chance to explain.

I didn't realize that I was afraid of him until this morning when I hung up the phone and told my wife my plan to drive three hours south today.

I said to her, "It's a weird thing. I'm angry and I'm sad—sad for myself and for my father. But it's all been secret and private."

"Your father's dying was the major event of your life," she said, "Other than meeting me."

I smiled, but I was afraid to the point of collapse.

"Oh, go ahead and meet him," she said. "You like explanations. You and Gresser have been silently colluding for years. He's made you who you are. You might as well talk to him. If you come back sadder and angrier, it happens. I'll rub your neck."

She put her hand on my shoulder, steadied me.

She knew it would be a long day. Then she found for me part of a Frank Bidart poem.

> The love I've known is the love
> of two people staring
> not at each other, but in the same direction.

She smiled when she read it. She knew this was how I think of medicine.

Sometimes I think about the temporary disturbances in our ten years of marriage and how it's not all been splendid leisure. My wife has taken my distress and distance over the past ninety-six hours in good faith. She knows the state I'm in, although not all the reasons. She won't be drawn into my self-pity. Before I left for work and Gresser, she put in my bag a newspaper advertisement for a support group called Emotions Anonymous which I have just found: "If you want to live in serenity with unsolved problems, join us. 863-5555." My wife wrote *Hah!* on the bottom.

PART TWO

ON THIS FIRST day of June, Monday, I find George Dittus combing his hair in front of the television that is mounted from the ceiling in the patient social area on 9A. The open room, opposite the elevators, has a few overly soft, armless green couches that look as if they have been taken from the lobby of a hunting lodge. Although our hospital went smoke-free eighteen months earlier, the atmosphere still smells of cigarettes. When I say, "Mr. Dittus?" he turns to me, rises on his toes like a demagogue and says, "I need to get home." He has a stain in the crotch of his pajama pants and his ears are like the chewed ends of erasers. He has brass-colored hair that used to be bright red. He looks to be in his mid-fifties. At six-feet or so, he is just about my size, but he looks like he hasn't gotten any sun in a decade.

Whenever I am on 9A I take the opportunity to stand for a moment in this lounge to look out the window beyond the TV, over the interstate, over the river and the parked tug that never helped anyone, to the nineteenth-century houses that come down to the water from College Hill. This Monday though, I mostly stare at Mr. Dittus.

"I think I got one of those letters that say 'You may already have won a free trip to Aruba," he says to me.

What do I know from his second sentence? I am as judgemental as any; I figure he is a joker. He has been watching the lounge TV, Ed McMahon has come on with his bulk mail tease, and Mr. Dittus is offering it to me as a test. Patients are always testing me in one way or another, offering me their arcane enthusiasms or fears, trusting that I follow their logic. And I'm making cascades of decisions. I do believe that he wants to get home.

Patients make me think of books and books make me think of patients; the association allows me to enjoy both a bit more. This day I think of *The Travels of Marco Polo*, which I finished a few weeks back. When Marco visits the Great Khan, the khan's emissaries have recently returned and they render an account of their mission but give no other report of the countries they visit. The khan declares that he would rather "hear reports of these strange countries and of their customs and usages than the business on which he sent them." My business is medicine, and I have the sense immediately that Mr. Dittus is a strange country. At this first meeting I can't place George Dittus, but I have the sense that I have met him before.

•

My doctoring is unusual, I've been told, although to my mind, the unconventional doctor has become something of a convention. The typical unconventional doctor shocks patients, in voice, in manner, in attitude. The truly unusual doctor lets patients shock him. 'Say anything to me. I can take it.' That's my motto. My wife, who thinks that I'm unusual, who will also say anything to me ("Odd. You're odd," she told me recently), quoted Hemingway to me on our first date. We were watching the Celtics whip the Bullets in my living room. She was wearing pearls and cowboy boots and she said, "The world breaks everyone and afterward many are strong in the broken places." I don't remember exactly what we were talking about, but she said that and it went to my head.

My wife knows everything about me, every secret, things I would rather keep to myself but can't because of her green eyes and the way that she bites down on my ribs when we're playing and she senses that I have something to say. She knows almost nothing about medicine although doctors assume she does because she's married to a doctor. Luckily, she has a sense of humor.

She knows that I take care of about fifteen hospitalized patients during these months that I work "on the wards." This rotating fifteen (they come and go, discharges, new arrivals) are "ward" patients because they had no regular doctor when they suddenly became ill and arrived at the emergency room, or because they had a doctor who did not admit patients to my hospital where an ambulance brought them for various reasons—the hospital the patient preferred was full, or there was too much traffic going that way and the ambulance driver wasn't in the mood to flash his lights—or because they were simply people visiting from out of town who got sick. This triage leads to a compelling mixture on my "ward"—the homeless to the luxury-homed. When I say that I take care of these patients, I mean that the medical students, interns and residents who are indentured to me, my team, "takes care of" them, because I work in a teaching hospital. My team does the first wave medical work; they draw the blood, do the first examination (the nurses actually perform ninety percent of the hospital's functions and probably spend the most satisfying time with patients), and I offer critical appreciation. This "team" concept adds an athletic overtone to my day, but the men and women who make up my team don't blink at being called a team, the whole bunch of them cut-throat and competitive since grade school.

A good part of my day involves the indigent and this puts me high on an unspoken liberal hierarchy. It makes me virtuous and generally above reproach—at least professionally—among acquaintances. The whole old, noble profession of medicine used to be thought of in this awestruck way, but now the snake on the staff is just a snake and proof has to be offered as to your do-good status. Of course, most people do not think of the fact that the poor don't sue and are often also frankly grateful, unlike the not-so-poor, so really I am a different and easier sort of opportunist. I have created a schedule that allows time to read most anything that comes across my desk, to look out my window, to enjoy, on lazy days, a progressive unreality. Not a bad life.

Last night I started reading Julian Barnes' *Flaubert's Parrot*, a book about the life and times of that great author, and I came across the following sentence: "Medicine then must have been a exciting, desperate, violent business; nowadays it is all pills and bureaucracy."

While I have no doubt that hospitals reflect their times

just as novelists do, I thought that Barnes had gotten it quite wrong. In fact, I have always thought that where I work is a place of great occasions. I don't mean great in the sense of happy, of course. No one is happy in the hospital. Even when patients are about to leave they still have head-scratching concerns about causes and repeat episodes. I mean great in the sense of special, in the sense of trembly momentous.

Yes, there are the eccentric minor characters who seem made for sitcoms, and there are many rules because non-sense often demands precision, and there are certainly pills by the fistful. But the yearning sadness, the strange mix of satire and elegy are what matter in the hospital.

When I studied piano, I despised sight-reading. I had no skill for it and I lived in fear of those weeks when my teacher would open in front of me a score I had never seen before. I became frustrated almost immediately. Rummaging for notes humiliated me.

After all, I had practiced and prepared, and she had me trying to make music from fingerings I didn't know, and I felt, during these lessons, that my teacher had a particular fondness for my undoing.

After I quit piano, claiming too many fingers broken at sports, I did not experience that lost and awkward feeling of sight-reading again until I saw patients. Again, I could blame only my ignorance and incompetence.

A small part of medicine is pills and a large part is meet-ing patients like George Dittus. I know that I will be seeing a lot of George, but I need to include other things as well here, even bleak and violent things. What I want to explain to myself is the dilating space of a person's history, how it's both troubling and something to be thankful for.

I'm superstitious sometimes. I believe in the big and unanswerable. I respect peoples' definition of their illnesses and have considered the incongruity of a thirty-five-year-old telling his elders what's what.

Barnes was being sentimental. I see medicine in Flaubert's time as an abandoned cabin in the forest, a pathetic but well-preserved ruin. While there may be some pills and bureaucracy nowadays, there is very little that is sentimental.

•

Here is a list of the patients whom I see on the day that Mr. Dittus comes in. One is knitting an afghan during her stay for pneumonia, one is part Cherokee and demented, another is so fat she couldn't make it to the bathroom or onto a bedpan so her daughter put newspapers on the floor around her bed and she just rolled over to the edge and went; she is admitted with phlebitis. I ask another, a ninety-year-old man with anemia what his happiest memory is (a light, non-medical question meant to stir conversation), and he tells me it was when he was a boy living in his parents' home; there hasn't been much good since. The rest of my patients are international: a woman basketball coach with high blood pressure who fled Azerbaijan, a dizzy lady from Laos, a man from Puerto Rico whose kidneys had stopped. Old clam-colored men, women with hair buns like hand-grenades.

My city is like so many others, in recession, with lousy grade schools and ambitious little madmen, thieves really, running City Hall, gathering pensions, stealing from credit unions. After ten years here, I wouldn't live anywhere else. My hometown supplies more than enough customers for ward 9A. I think of 9A as one street, one neighborhood, of the second city I live in and love, my hospital.

The city of the hospital is not often seen in the way it needs to be seen. Like all cities it is a place of violence and menace and incessant noise and tough, dark pride. It is filled with workers who stir respect. Each moment, for those of us who work here, there are a thousand new sensations. Most visitors avert or otherwise occupy their eyes, swarmed by the traffic of The White Life. For them, there are functions to perform, relatives to embrace, the move-ment of sympathy, and so visitors only glance at surfaces, always a little afraid. Those who live in the city, staff and patients, see more and are bothered less.

I ask Mr. Dittus to come with me back to his room where we can speak privately. The television in the patient lounge has no off button and as we stroll away, side by side, I hear a commercial that begins, "Do you know what malpractice is?" and I turn to put a face with this message, a message I never imagined would be able to penetrate the walls of a hospital, that would be invisibly censored. The man has a well-scrubbed face, a dark blue suit, almost no make-up, one of those local, amateur-studio, lusty-with-ambition performances. Mr. Tooth-for-a-Tooth.

I think I hear Mr. Dittus chuckle, but perhaps he is only clearing his throat. He's skinny and soft at the same time, not a bit youthful, with unhappy teeth spaced unevenly by decay.

We take a few steps and he is up on his toes again. His toes are in green hospital slippers.

"I'm ready to go home," he says.

"Mr. Dittus, I don't even know why you're here," I say. I haven't read his chart yet or spoken to my team.

"I think I'm ready."

"Perhaps you are, but why don't you let me have a few words with you first."

"I feel fine. No point in staying."

"Stay a little while," I say, without knowing anything about him or how long he would need to stay or even why I am bargaining with a patient I've met only two minutes before.

"I just want to get to my own house." His eyes bob and weave; they're hard to locate.

"When you're ready, I'll be the first to get you out of here," I tell him.

"I'm ready."

I try to be calm, nonchalant, neutral. No promises.

I am not ready to let him leave; he cannot leave safely. I do not send people home just because they ask.

He turns and walks toward his room.

An antlered deer estimated to weigh 265 pounds crashed through a window of our hospital last month. In our small state, the city is not far from the suburban woods and the buck was determined to get inside. He went for the plate-glass.

He was apparently in rut. When he saw his reflection, he must have thought he was seeing another male and attacked. When he had battered his way inside, he butted a wall mural depicting a forest before getting trapped in the engineering department offices, tearing up the place, cut and bleeding. It was the middle of the day and the staff boarded up the smashed window and dimmed the lights in an effort to calm the deer.

A conservation officer arrived with PVC pipe and copper tubing and blew two tranquilizer darts into the deer, avoiding a powder-charged gun that would have been loud and risked ricochet.

The buck was treated for lacerations and contusions in our emergency room. The staff was somber, perhaps taking the attack as an omen. When the deer was patched up, he was loaded onto a stretcher, carried to a truck, and driven the half-mile out of the city where he was laid on some leaves and watched over until he shook himself awake and walked into the woods.

Knowing when to send the patient home is a doctor's job.

•

When a patient and doctor move through the halls together, looks from other patients fall into two categories. There are those stares that are envious; these two know each other well and my doctor knows nothing about me. And there are jabbing eyes that quickly look away, back to the TV, out the window at the highway, the river, the smokestacks, the clapboard houses; that doc has bad news for him, it's his last happy walk, poor sucker.

The hall on 9A is white-walled with a wide wooden

hand-rail at hip height. You can't walk this twenty-yard stretch in a straight line. There are laundry hampers and drug carts and scales and chairs in the way. There are walkers without walkees and stepping stools and gurneys with people getting wheeled to tests. Sometimes there are drips of blood, or tracks a boot (hexagram style) has left like a hopscotch board. I have never seen a hospital hall without obstacles. Our hospital is shaped like a boomerang with an elevator shaft at the curve, 9A at one end, 9B at the other. I make wide arcs around the rooms that smell of urine or vomit, the unreasonable affairs of mortals, smells I have never gotten used to although they are as familiar as photos on a desk. Usually, when I stop to speak with someone, I lean against the walls that I know are warm; the walls of hospitals are always warm.

Mr. Dittus walks back to his room with his head down, smelling his neck, hunched, that attitude. In fact, I have no bad news for Mr. Dittus; I only want to hear why he has come to the hospital.

I walk miles in a day. Room to room. When I come to a halt, I can't stop walking. I stand shifting from one foot to the other. When I walk it is not leisurely; I am not strolling. There's always a distraction: another patient who wants to see me, a nurse with a suggestion, a colleague who wants to chat. There's the noise of the showers. Hospital showers are loud: firm spray on tile behind wooden doors. A booming and an echoing. Patients don't even hear me when I knock.

There is noise summoning me from everywhere. In the wild, loud noises connote danger. I've been told by patients that I scream when I mean to speak in a normal voice. Noise cancellation technology has been developed, I've read. Digitally synthesized, out-of-phase anti-noise cancels the alarms, the hydraulic door checks, the gears of rising beds that fill hospitals. What would this be like? The hospital where I now work could be any I have ever worked in. There's a familiarity. There are associations, even with the noise. Looking into patient rooms makes me think of other patients.

health. I think of the horrendous month I spent on crutches as a ten-year-old after falling from a jungle gym. My mother believes that walks can cure anything, a cold, boredom, a bad marriage. She walks a mile a day. Walking is our natural rhythm, the rhythm of health. It is a hopeful rhythm; maybe the verticality is as important as the movement. When I walk with an old patient down the halls it reminds me of walks I took with my father during which we spoke most intimately.

Many of the sick whom I care for cannot walk. They are not vertical and therefore are not hopeful. I once worked in a hospital that regularly built additions, a wing here, a new clinic there. I had a patient with a stroke who had not yet risen from bed. When he saw the building going up outside his window, he was reassured. The building was vertical, walking. Propped up, he would wave at the men in their boots on the scaffolding and they would wave back at him.

When patients improve, part of their improvement often involves walking. My uncle who lives in the country says, "When the step is ahead of the thought, the mind can wander." Walking in the woods brings on contemplation. Here, the sick have to think, have to remember how to walk. They move straight ahead first; they do not zigzag or jump the cracks in the floor, the games of children. Walking still stirs thinking but the thoughts are sad ones, of grandchildren that will no longer be easily carried, of beaches that will never be visited again. I once worked with a doctor who could not rise from his wheelchair. Everyone trusted him; for patients he was like looking in the mirror.

As we pass, some would think that George Dittus is not particularly sick because he can walk as well as the doctor beside him. On the way to his room, he uses walking as evidence that he is not sick, although he favors his right foot I notice.

"My legs are strong, Doc. Strong," he tells me.

"No doubt," I say.

•

25

My hospital has its own light and time and smells and sounds. Like other cities it has sections—business districts, supply outlets, markets where people mingle. There are city services: mail delivery, public (patient) transportation, carpentry. All the processes that make up the life of a city— creation, damage, decay, rehabilitation, removal—correspond to life in the hospital. Large hospitals have not only been built in inner cities, they have become their own urban centers.

A sunny day has become cloudy and the color of the 9A hall has changed. All cities have their own peculiar light. Provincetown's cobalt morning, Jerusalem's dry white reflections, Cairo's dust. Hospital light is impossible light, chronic light, a constant effect that seems hardly a light at all.

During the day, no one notices the glow. On the ninth floor, eyes are drawn to the windows in each room, to the fast clouds white as parchment, to the pigeons gurgling on ledges, gulls circling, lemon-rind sun coming through the streaky glass, through even the wide tan shades. You wouldn't even know the lights were on. But at night, when the windows are black, the light inside continues, illuminating what's there to be known. It is always day in the hospital, someone always needs to see and be seen. If a bulb flickers in a hall, all limbs on the ward seem to shake. Otherwise, it is ordinary, straight light in high wattage: shadowless. There are no distortions or transformation, no soft surfaces, no brilliance, iridescence, splendor.

In the rooms, there are no fringed lamps, no tiny plug-in Mickey Mouse night light. Beds are back-lit by thin bulbs hidden behind faux wood. This weak light seems to slide down along the wall. The light in each room is the same.

Every day in the conference room at the end of the ward, I put X-rays up to another light looking for fractures, the slaughter of organs. Illumination comes through the body. Penetrates. The body glows.

When I was a third-year medical student, I participated

26

in open heart surgery under the brilliant lights of the operating room. When the patient's chest was open, the surgeon
asked if I wanted to feel the living beating heart. As I
touched it with great gentleness, the lights went out in the
room. A power failure. In the startling darkness, my hand
on the heart, I felt a great calm and I remained still for what
seemed a long time. In the dark, the person below me whose
heart I held was protected. Above that open chest, I imagined steam rising from a lake, I don't know why. The back-
up generator went on. Then there was light.

•

I have the sense that Mr. Dittus is bereft of something,
something he probably never had, and which maybe I can
give him. He sits on a bed which sinks in the middle, and I
sit beside him on what looks like an Adirondack chair with
mustard yellow cushions that hiss as I land. I move forward,
trying to act thoughtful and likable (although I have an
inbred pessimism), but keep slipping back. On closer
inspection, I see that Mr. Dittus's reddish hair is brushed
back off his high forehead, which brings out those troubled
ears. His eyes are asymmetric, the right slightly lower than
the left, and brown. He has not shaved in days and his nails
have been neglected. He looks like the owner of a second-
hand bookstore.

I call him by his last name here as a formality, although
it is not how I think of him. I know that within a few days I
will be using his first name without asking if this is what he
prefers. This is wrong, I know; I should always ask what
patients prefer rather than assuming intimacy; but I don't; I
see it as my prerogative although, arguably, a disrepectful
one. With some people, of course, I never use their first
name: they will always be Mr. Pontorellis or Mrs.
Handmans, just as when you grow up there are still parents
in the neighborhood who remain Mister and Missus rather
than Brad and Lillian. First names in the hospital are like
nicknames, signs of affection. The nurses always call

patients by their first names. They just walk in and say Hello, Gladys, and nobody blinks.

I forget to close the pale blue curtain that runs along the ceiling around his bed, and I have to stand again with another hiss and tug its skimpy material along the rungs. One rusty runner catches and there I am jerking at it in a fly-fishing spasm as Mr. Dittus's roommates stare at me. Once this is done, we have a kind of privacy although there are still three other patients in their beds within our fifteen-by-twenty-foot room. (Our hospital is medieval in many ways, one of which is still having four-bed rooms). With the curtain closed, our space becomes a little darker and the confinement pushes my chair closer to his bed. The curtain becomes a door, a window, and the outline of a new room. The pulling of the thin blue curtains fools no one; everyone can still hear us, but it makes those outside matter less. It is the first tacit agreement we make, me and Mr. Dittus; we both know the world will go on but we won't talk about it within our curtain. The voices out there might as well be birds. No one can see us.

•

Doctors are primarily information gatherers and in many ways like spies. We must work backwards, often without all the facts. We trade in secrets and whispers, and we are dependent on what we are told; this makes us impatient. My wife has pointed out to me that studies reveal we most often interrupt our patients within twenty seconds of starting an interview. Knowing this, I am cautious and content to keep quiet.

"I'm out front washing my car when I get this feeling in my chest. Like last time. I'm doing circles with my rag and it's getting heavier and heavier," George Dittus tells me. His right arm is stirring the soup of air between us. "So they told me when I went home if this pain came back I should come back. I went home two weeks ago. I told all this already."

He had indeed, although not to me. Chest pain has been

his entry ticket in the emergency room, a common enough complaint, often used by those who know the system, who know how to use it to get indoors on a cold, homeless day. The easiest way into a hospital for a man his age.

Every male doctor I know is scared of having a heart attack himself. As the joke between us goes: Question: What do you do if someone comes into your office, you give them a clean bill of health and send them on their way only to have them die on the path in front of your building? Answer: You turn them around.

"You were last here when?" I ask George, disturbed.

When he repeats "two weeks ago," I think: I must have passed him in the halls when he was here last month. That's why he looks familiar to me. But this possibility doesn't explain why the conversation we're having feels so important, why I'm listening so carefully.

"They don't tell you very much, do they?" he says. "You must be in charge."

In my mustard chair I think: Yes, I'm the one in charge. My name is the one on your bracelet. The bracelets have always seemed odd to me. They remind me of the tagging of animals on National Geographic television specials, animals dart-gunned, marked, and tracked across continents.

Looking at George's bracelet makes me reach into my pocket to check the index card I keep there that has been stamped with the same information that appears on Mr. Dittus's bracelet. This morning, I found a pack of these index cards stuck to my office door, the outer one V-ed to enfold approximately ten others, each with a purple-inked name on it.

This pack of index cards represents my ward patients who have been admitted to the hospital by an unfortunate colleague who was working the weekend. The cards are left hanging in a pharmaceutical toy, magnetized to my door and extending its card-holder grip with a big, drug company name. Purists, of course, would not allow this object or any related to it—pen, pad, coffee mug—near their office; such free drug company advertising implies the coopting and

29

bribing of someone who now only made their weakness public. It is true that every so often I do clean my office of these knick-knacks, and I bring them home to my wife and children who collect and enjoy them as signs of my sins; they already know me as someone who favored disposable diapers, someone easily corporately tampered with.

My thumb always becomes purple carrying this stack of cards. My wife inevitably sees this discoloration on my finger at home in the evening and wonders for a moment whether it is blood, questioning the adequacy of my glove-use and hand-washing.

I keep only a few notes about the patients on these index cards; late in the day they are generally useless because I often can not read what I have written; this has been a problem since my earliest school days. The cards fit in my shirt pocket. The purple-inked inscription holds a whole life of information: the admitting doctor's name (me), the patient's name, date of birth. Religion comes as a three-letter computer-useful mouthful: BAP for Baptist, PSB for Presbyterian, RMC for Roman Catholic. Sometimes there is UNK in this space (Mr. Dittus has UNK) and I feel a special protective sense for these persons because UNK means: (1) they were too sick to tell their religion and had arrived with no relatives or friends who could offer help, or (2) they refused to get involved with a question that could lead to all sorts of assumptions—priestly visits on weekdays, special rites, etc., or (3) an unlucky and potentially forboding transcription error had occurred down in the Admitting Office.

I take Mr. Dittus's card out of my pocket to write some notes as I say to him, "Tell me more about your chest pain."

•

Mr. Dittus arrives without having a regular doctor he calls his own. We, who provide care, must therefore learn about him from scratch. Both he and I come to the encounter slightly distrustful, scanning, making calculations, hopeful.

I watch a lot of television at home and doctoring is like

TV. It's all close-ups. I believe that there is an excess of close-ups; there is rarely time to step back. But Mr. Dittus is amazingly composed, peaceful even, and somehow, on this Monday, it makes me step back. I don't often bring work home, certainly not any mental work. But there are times when particular patients just occur to me; when I am doing the dishes or tossing in the laundry. Or when I'm reading. And at work when certain patients come to mind, so do things I have recently read.

Looking at George Dittus brings to mind what the poet Jack Gilbert writes:

> When the King of Siam disliked a courtier,
> he gave him a beautiful white elephant.
> The miracle beast deserved such ritual
> that to care for him properly meant ruin.
> Yet to care for him improperly was worse.
> It appears the gift could not be refused.

•

This sense of meeting someone whom I've met before—which I experienced immediately with George Dittus—must be a sign of reaching a particular stage in life, for it's happened several times in the last few months. My memory is beginning to fade at the very time the remembered past has become an important source of pleasure for me.

Not long ago I worked with a medical student, a woman nearly fifteen years younger than I am, whom I found myself staring at in the halls. She was a lovely woman with short blonde hair, long thin arms, and perfect, muscular veins on her hands. Although she had just become my student, I had a hard time convincing myself that we hadn't been introduced some years before. I felt that I knew the way her heavy sweater slid up from her wrist. When I studied her from a distance, it produced a unique anxiety, and drove me a little crazy. But she gave no sign that she recognized me. I was attracted to her (as I do not allow with most students), but more than that, when we separated after a few minutes of standard student-teacher conversation, I felt a loneliness, like the stir of early romance, which I knew had little to do with her. At the end of our second day together, I asked her if we had ever met before and she assured me that we had not.

On the fourth day of her rotation, I realized that she reminded me of my first girlfriend, Renata, with whom I once spent a lot of time in the cool dark. When I made this connection—Renata also had beautiful arms and long, thin fingers—my student began to disappoint me (before my reason returned). She did not answer the way Renata would have answered; she had slimmer hips; she did not look at me in the way I remembered Renata had.

•

"Pain," George says again, "right here."

I ask for his unprompted description, knowing full well that ordinary experience (let alone pain) is sometimes hopelessly beyond anyone's power to describe and beyond my power to analyze. I push him because that's what I was taught medicine is: an assembly of names and facts. There is a harm to this attitude and I feel it within seconds. Already my relation with Mr. Dittus has become purposive, always seeking greater knowledge. This is dreadfully serious—within seconds it has become a duty, a school lesson. But to think of this conversation otherwise, that I might be sitting here trying to evoke emotion in Mr. Dittus, or perhaps, if his pain were gone, to think of more pleasant things with him, seems childish, frivolous, and I would be like the author of those eighteenth-century scientific treatises who, right in the middle of a closely-reasoned discussion of physiology, includes a quote from Cicero, ruining our serious modern reading. Such an interpolation simply seems too personal.

"You were here, in this hospital, two weeks ago?"

"Same thing. Pain, here," he thumps his chest. "But last time, the senior guy got here first. That's strange, don't you think?"

When I start to take the history of his pain I am trying to trip him up. That's my strategy. If I get him to say a few key words I can convince myself that this chest pain has nothing to do with his heart. Maybe one of the other organs in there is acting up, some body part not doing its job. The regular ferocious sucking, the downdrafts of fluid, the ballooning and submarining innards of an organ *other* than the heart is just off a bit. Is it really pain or do you really mean—and here I've always wanted to offer some options taken from the natural world, a wobble, a trill, a keening, that might better represent that pain (but I never offer)—do you really mean discomfort? Yeah, that's it, do you really mean discomfort? Because while pain probably means something bad, discomfort more likely means something not so bad. I want to trip him up so I can convince myself that it isn't going to be bad for Mr. Dittus. Then I can move on to the more important facts like when he will go home and when I will go home (or at least on to my fourteen other waiting patients).

•

It seems odd that someone down in the emergency room had decided that Mr. Dittus's pain did not signal a serious cardiac problem, and had sent him to 9A rather than to Intensive Care. That he had been here with the same problem two weeks before (I didn't yet have his medical record to tell me the details of that admission) is concerning. But instead of making the simple assumption that someone in the Emergency Room had been depressingly lax in their triage, I make the opposite assumption: Mr. Dittus is a crank.

When he says to me, "I told all this already," I know it is a bother for him to tell it again. He keeps stumbling— "It just hurt," "It was like an electric frying pan," "Haven't you ever felt pain in your chest?"—until something about Mr. Dittus makes me suddenly abandon the suspended, circling rhythm of these questions and I ask him what kind of car he drives. His car, after all, had been the only witness to his chest pain. I wonder if someone else hearing this change of direction in our talk might find the same use in it that I do or would simply think of me as insane. Specifically, what would my students think of my follow-up questions about how long he's owned his car, what kind of wax he uses on it, how many miles it has, what the longest trip he's ever taken in it is.

I was sent a series of essays last week by a former student of mine who left medicine to study what he called, "the foundations of medical thinking." He had been sending me these small packages for about six months and I had watched his youthful professional ambition turn into piety for pure philosophy (this usually happens during the first year of college). In the latest installment, he included essays by "postmodernists, structuralists, who were working on durable problems that might be of interest." I knew by the time I'd read one of my former student's "impressions" that he had given up the incantations of medicine for an even more priestly variety and I felt bad for his wife who had three kids with her all day and no time for his dithering. Still, I read what he sent.

After I'd scanned a few of these essays, pacing, and after I'd quarrelled with myself for fifteen minutes, I wrote my student a short note pointing out that the "Foundations of Medical Thinking" spring from talking with patients and that there were actually only four things that mattered: (1) What you will say to them, (2) What you would like to say to them, (3) What you will feel when saying what you say and, (4) What the person in front of you will feel when you say it. "These four questions are the playground of medicine," I wrote, and "most everything else would seem comical" if he remembered only these four things.

Then I advised him what I had never advised anyone before: Go back to being a doctor.

These essays come to mind as I speak with Mr. Dittus

who seems more and more bored by the intellectual traps I am setting. What I would like to say to Mr. Dittus is: Hurry up and give me the facts. I'm busy; I have other patients to see. But I would feel unworthy saying this. Instead, I have developed a sophisticated way of moving quickly: I have cast him as an opponent (I keep asking, "What do you mean by that?"), an opposite team to be beaten. Me and my team of students against him. I find myself enjoying my challenges to him and when he answers me clearly, I am disappointed. The acquiring is more enjoyable than having acquired.

•

"Taking a history" is the phrase we doctors use for the initial interview with a patient. It is amazing how little life can be boiled down to if you're in a rush. The emphasis is usually on the "history," that enormous mix of circumstance and nature that we hear backwards. But let's consider the "taking." Whatever happened to Mr. Dittus that led him to the Emergency Room, we had taken and written in charts, printed on computer sheets, blown up on screens, by the time he reached 9A. In my thinking, I have taken his first and last names and replaced them with *Chest Pain*. The rest is just a story. On the way to 9A others had already revoked his wallet, his hat, his shoes. His things had been collected; *he* had been collected, like a beetle, in our compulsion to seek a new medical name for him. Our attitude toward the sick is not distinct from our attitude toward 'lesser life.'

"Chest pain," which is all I have actually written on my five-by-eight card after twenty minutes with him, makes me concentrate with detachment, released from confusion. The act of writing "Chest pain" is my version of using a microscope's eyepiece. It allows me to magnify form and shape, to single out. I feel near the essence of disease when I write it. But like a microscope's eyepiece, it also curtails the possibilities of seeing. It's correct only up to a point. Still, I gladly accept this paradox of medical language. After years at this job, I know about Chest Pain.

Dittus, despite the stain in the crotch of his pajama pants, smells sweet, like Portuguese bread. How exceptional this is: the typical runny smells of my job make me want to yell, "Try wiping yourself," as I walk these halls.

Only last year I learned how my hospital gets rid of these smells: we burn five million pounds of garbage a year. We don't dump; none of those contaminated, infectious syringes that turn up on beaches come from our hospital— they're ash around here. One hundred ninety one thousand pounds of empty cans, 654,000 pounds of cardboard, 147 pounds of plastic, 467,000 pounds of paper.

There are two old brick chimneys, each 150 feet tall right next to my office. They are quite impressive, beauteous even. Masoning bricks into tapering circles has always amazed me. The two puff out anything the incinerator offers, a steady stream of white smoke and ash. They look like very tall cannons.

If you ask Jimmy, the engineer who runs the incinerator to describe his machine he says, "It's thorough." The incinerator is in the basement of the main building (next to shipping and receiving, and the morgue) and looks like a printing press with its thrust and motor bearings, its valves, its damper linkages, air controls and fans.

"If you wanted to get rid of your wife, not even a finger would be left," Jimmy once said to me.

"Oh yeah?" I answered. Suddenly I knew what they talked about down there all day. Jimmy, looking at my smile, slowly understood what he had just said, and smiled himself.

"What I mean is, we do research animals, three-hundred-pound pigs."

Jimmy has a paunch and a gold chain. Wherever he puts his hand down, he leaves five black fingerprints.

"Not that your wife is a three hundred pound pig," he added.

Jimmy has learned to burn body parts (amputations, lab animals) only during the evening shift so that they burn all night. Even at 1700 degrees in a rotary kiln, you can't burn things too long, according to him. He learned the hard way, finding bits and pieces once after a quick flame. After that, he and his men started calling the incinerator the "spare parts machine."

•

There are courses for doctors who want to hone their interviewing skills. Until the invention of these courses, great skill in interviewing was assumed to derive naturally from attending medical school, from medical students seeing patients in the company of experienced doctors, and from watching these doctors track down the flawed, uncertain, elusive patient story. When the public rightly complained that doctors didn't know how to speak with them, that we interrupted and didn't listen, these courses took shape.

But as I speak with Mr. Dittus I come to believe yet again (as I did when I first heard of these courses) that our conversation is not teachable. For what is irreplaceable is his personality and my response to it, a response which includes the four questions I had mailed off to my former student. The learnable techniques in these courses could only provide an *imitation* or a *replica* of a good interview. It seems to me then that the formulae taught there are two-edged. They might enrich the skills of the participants in a vague, unchallengable way, but in some other way this enrichment is damaging. Telling people how and why and when they ought to feel is useful only in that it dispels a certain basic ignorance and remoteness that too many doctors have (although the worst offenders probably do not attend such courses); brought to the patient, this ignorance has a good chance of causing harm. But such courses as I'm describing do not allow self-discovery. You cannot teach people their own nature, their tastes. A patterned approach to interviews makes for egalitarianism, but Mr. Dittus is not the equal of my other patients.

By this I mean he owns a Rambler. Blue. One hundred forty thousand miles. Original engine. It seems to me a

good-hearted car, a car out of another era, a car that's both
an aberration on the road and a ballad to not keeping up-to-
date. It strikes me: George Dittus is a man out-of-place, and
this is endearing. I like old cars and I've generally liked the
people who drive them; they haven't capitulated, and they
have a little arrogance because of it.

He has taken one "long drive" years before to Boston,
forty-five miles north. "Where else would I go?" he asks
me; he has never been married and he lives alone. He tells
me that he has no living family. Not a one. He tells me that
he makes do off a Social Security check for $504 a month.

When I am leaving our curtained space he says, "You
know what the pain was like? It's like when you're cooking
spaghetti sauce and you haven't stirred it in a while and the
bottom of the pot is hot, and the top just has a few bubbles,
but it looks like the bubbles are sinking, like the top of the
sauce is collapsing. That's what the pain was like."

"Gassy," I say, probably missing the point, nearly mute
with familiarity with this complaint of chest pain which I
have heard a thousand times. I will hear "chest pain" a thousand times more and each time it will make its official way
to a medical record although it has a thousand meanings not
one of which is clear to me when I complete this conversation with Mr. Dittus.

I leave his room and head back to the coffee room next
to the nurses' station where I can jot a few thoughts about
Mr. Dittus in his medical record and also cadge some of the
food the nurses always leave around—popcorn, saltines,
brownies. Every coffee room now has a microwave (which
is different from the hot trays used when I was in training),
opening new reheating possibilities, such as lunches carried
out of the cafeteria and abandoned during a medical emergency so that scavengers like me could pick them over,
explaining later I thought they were just leftovers.

A nurse comes in behind me and asks, "Who did you
just see?"

"Mr. George Dittus," I tell her, trying to wedge the
saltines back into their packages.

"That guy won't stay in his bed," she says.

"He won't stay in bed," has a coded meaning: "he's a pain in the ass." It means: I'm really not much interested in being his nurse.

As at home, much of what happens in a hospital happens in bed. Sign-up for television service and telephone operation occurs there, as do most discussions with doctors. Nurses need their patients in bed at times to check vital signs and reset intravenous lines. Patients out of bed mean more work for the nurses who must interrupt their routine to find the missing person. But lying in bed in a hospital implies you're sick (at home you are just nestling) and so, the reluctance on the part of some to hang around their beds unless fixed there by wires or IVs or doctors' orders.

"I got him to sit down. I even talked to him," I tell her.

"Amazing," she says, shaking her head and walking out.

•

I must say that I do not like Mr. Dittus at first. He is not eloquent, preferring short answers; he is not at ease; he is impatient and touchy; and he is not obviously, obsequiously grateful to me. However, for reasons that are not yet apparent to me, I accept his obscurity as a virtue. Perhaps because he has a certain energy, and an obvious enthusiasm for his car despite the depressing ordeal of being in a hospital twice in one month.

Compared to the thirty-seven-year-old nurse who has also been admitted to 9A over the weekend after fainting, I do not like George Dittus at all. She is about my age, knows as much about hospitals as I do, knows she does not want to be here except to be doing her job (she works in the outpatient endocrinology clinic), knows that she wants to see a cardiologist in addition to me (similar to many health professionals she has no doctor of her own other than a gynecologist who works only below the belt). She is much braver than I would have been, but her husband is a wreck, sweaty and bald, and for that I like her also. He is sitting on her bed when I come in. She is sitting on top of the covers, heart monitors under her robe. Patient autonomy is directly proportional to the number of clothes a patient wears that they own, and she has come prepared. She has a satchel that, lying flat, zips up like a smile.

I don't call her by her first or her last name. I don't say her name at all when I introduce myself. Saying her name might bring bad luck. I give her my first and last names. She's had palpitations for years, and slowly cut out coffee, chocolate, liquor (all those things that, when avoided, might not actually help you live longer but would certainly made you feel like you had). Her attacks are more frequent during periods of stress; she had once tried a medicine to decrease their severity, eventually giving that up as a failure. She functioned quite well until she hit the ground, waking up on her green living room rug Sunday morning. Saturday, she had had a long dizzy period with her heart pounding, without fainting, but this was the first real faint.

What do I do for her that is special? When we speak I give her as much time as she needs, I do not rush her. I call the cardiologist to *hear* his opinion rather than read it in the chart, and I translate his description of the available options into language that is useful to her. When she asks me about the result of a specific blood test, and I don't know the answer, I walk out of the room and return immediately with the answer. I call technicians around the hospital to have her tests moved up on schedules so she can leave more quickly. I visit her twice a day rather than my usual single visit. I help her find her slippers which have slipped under the bed. I calm her husband who tells me that he doesn't even like sitting next to doctors, a comment I usually would have little tolerance for. Within twelve hours of her arrival, we find out that a hospital fifty miles away has the ability to do a sophisticated study we can't do here, and so we send her away for the best possible treatment. Back in my office, when I turn in my five-by-eight card with her name on it (the card goes to billing so I can get paid), my secretary calls me to say that I have written no diagnosis on it. I must not believe that she was actually sick.

Compared with my immediate and understandable feeling of closeness to this nurse, Mr. Dittus remains a stranger. When I say I am "close" to someone, I may not mean physical proximity; when I say someone is "far out" I may mean several things, not one of which has to do with location. I never closed the blue curtain around this nurse who also sat in a four-bed room. When I pull in close to Mr. Dittus's bed, I am both near and far. The term stranger has a spatial sense to it at times. I share no kinship with Mr. Dittus, no occupation, no common idiom. With my nurse I shared some of these, which may help to explain my immediate interest in her and why I treated her differently. I was a local, she was a local.

The hospital is a place of strangers and a place for strangers. So when I asked Mr. Dittus about his car, which I did quite naturally, without hesitation, I was trying to translate him into a familiar; I drive a Ford now but I remember my first car, a yellow Volkswagen that cost me preposterous repair bills which I gladly paid as it aged and rattled, a car that I eventually sold (under pressure from my wife who was tired of rescuing me when it stopped mid-highway) just at a time when my hair loss was accelerating, a sickening linkage in my mind that disturbs me still.

There is nothing special about turning strangers into manageable guests. It happens everywhere, even outside hospitals, but *how* this is done makes all the difference. In the hospital, our claim is that whatever we do for the stranger is for *his good.* There is a clash, an inevitable incongruity, between the good of my patients and my own good. I have already described when I wrote about how I first considered Mr. Dittus's chest pain, I wanted to convince myself that it was not heart-derived so that I could move on to the next patient, leaving him with a still-undefined pain, pain with a question mark. Publicly, that is to students who await my opinions eagerly (this eagerness earns them good evaluations they hope), our care is efficient and technically correct if a person leaves feeling better than when they arrived, even if every question, such as the origin of their chest pain, has not been answered.

Mr. Dittus is a stranger, but he is also a guest, a hospital guest. The echo chamber of words is helpful here: hospital, hostel, hotel; a lodging for strangers. He is a guest in my daily house, unexpected and unannounced, but a guest whom I approach with some *manners*, that wobbly word between rejection (as with the homeless in the emergency room) and immediate embracing (as with my nurse).

When Mr. Dittus said to me, "Two weeks ago, the senior guy got here first. *That's strange, don't you think?*" what he meant was: your hospital way is strange. And I believe him, yes, we must appear sublimely strange.

•

Sometimes I talk to my wife about Gresser. Not very often, but the last time I did she said, "It's like you're in this cult. The cult of Gresser. You're obsessed."

"A cult of one," I answered. "And I recruited myself."

It's a strange cult (although I'm sure many adults who lost a parent at a young age are also in such cults), and I don't feel part of it all the time. Most times I can grin at the horrible humor of someone my age not moving past this. Other times I feel taken over and pressured by my thoughts of Gresser. It's not a good thing.

How do you get out of a cult? The leader dies; you die; your family comes to save you. In this case, my mother won't rescue me and my father can't. Just as I couldn't save him.

Like most cultists, I'm happy with my life. Two sons who run around naked in the June heat, Coleman Hawkins on tape, my bedroom up in the trees, cool sheets, sunlight until 8:00 PM, my wife in an old white nightgown that fits loosely.

•

I live on the edge of the uncontrollable—crime, drugs, disease—but it is in the hospital that the wheel of the unanswerable stops in front of me. I have never met a patient who did not think they were immortal until the very end. Only then, the imagination surrenders itself to principle. The obsessive question that went round and round, the question left from childhood—"Am I going to die?"—stops. No one can prepare for their end, which is why I feel that every death I watch is an assassination.

On one wall of my office is the photograph of a tattooed man, his back bent like an oarsman so that I can see the tattoos covering his entire surface, abdomen, spine, arms to the wrists, legs, and I imagine him in the water like a trout, the inks flaring off of him as he swims trailing lines of color. At times this is how I think of medicine, patients slipping away, leaving vapors.

What I like about George springs from my interest in people who don't understand the rules, who don't understand what's happening to them, to their lives, who are confused by the signposts around them.

George and I are comparable in this way.

On my way to lunch it strikes me, the connection, the simple equation. The way his tongue moved against the inside of his cheek signalling impatience, the way I could trace its subterranean speed and direction (like the roaming of an eye under its lid in sleep), the way it passed between George Dittus' lips and teeth made me think of my father. A small but telling similarity, this gesture opened my eyes to the simple truth which had amazingly until then escaped my consciousness. Resemblance is really an imagined presence, and Mr. Dittus makes me feel as if my father were around again. Other signs come to me as confirmation: they both had red hair; they both sneered in condescension. They carried their hands the same way, slightly away from the body, when they walked.

I pass my father's portrait every morning when I'm in our family room putting *Sesame Street* back on for my children. While I've been out of the room (getting their clothes, packing their lunches), they've clicked over to Nickelodeon, ignoring my request to watch only public television, and when I return they giggle, and my father looks on.

When I study him I don't think of his death first-off; he is, after all, a man in his thirties above the mantel, red-headed and clean-shaven. But inevitably I do think of that last night. You'd think that twenty years downstream with a family of my own would mean enough is enough. But it's not. I don't stand and stare and mope like a traveler to Italy looks at his favorite saint—my children are in the room— but there's a startling sureness to my daily visit to this spot: my father's portrait and a thought of Gresser.

I don't feel morbid either. My thoughts lead to a strange twinge of resentment. My mother and Gresser were the only ones to see my father that last night. I need information from them, sometimes I feel as if I'm chasing them. My mother doesn't like to talk about it. "Ancient history," she says.

•

I have lunch with my dear friend David who has recently moved in with a doctor; they are each considering the prospects of a second marriage. He also has had fainting spells (perhaps another reason for my immediately liking that nurse) for the past few years, one or two a year that began with a wooziness, and proceeded to a slow graying out at unpredictable times. Once this had happened when driving and he had the time and brains to get off the road, park and faint. When he awoke a few minutes later, he drove himself in for consultation. The doctors I found him got no useful information from the tests they performed (David said he never was good at tests), and offered him no answers. When he had asked my opinion about the black-outs, I said nothing intelligent. His new friend, Liz, had sent him on a new round of tests through her doctor friends and he had ended up with a pacemaker under the broad flap of one pectoral as a preventative against the one faint that didn't end. (He once told me that he wanted his tombstone to read: I may be gone for some time.) This was our first time together since his surgery.

I make the mistake of saying something about how I get to see these amazing things everyday and who else gets to watch what I do, and shouldn't I be distilling some sort of meaning from all this life experience?

"Hah!" he hoots. David has small eyes and a big chest. "What do you know about doctors. You *are* a doctor."

He says, "My God, you're talking as if this work you do is the first and last honorable passion of man. Which it is for Liz, who works too hard and is actually useful in a way, but you?" And he gives me his big smile and pulls at his underbeard.

I am silent.

"Only patients learn things," David says. "At least tell me about your own experiences as a patient if you want to keep my interest at all."

"I've had none," I tell him.

"That's fascinating. You're quite a story-teller."

"No. Wait a minute. I broke my leg once and spent a night in an upstate New York infirmary trying to avoid having the nurses see up my gown and maneuvering onto a blue bedpan with a cast up to my hip."

"Unendingly amusing, even laudable," he says.

I have no tales of surgical sponges left in my abdomen, I have no strange under-anaesthesia experiences. But I realize at this meal with David twent-six years after my leg-break, the absurdity of my having been hospitalized back then, and the fact that such an overnight would never happen these days. With a broken leg now you'd barely get to see a doctor, intercepted instead by para-doctor levels, such as physicians' assistants and nurse practitioners who could do the same work, cheap labor. When my nephew recently broke his leg flying off a swing, my sister-in-law *insisted* that he see a doctor each visit and their orthopedist had no shame in charging $300 to remove the cast at the final visit, a procedure that took approximately fifteen seconds and could have been done by her husband who is a contractor with perfectly good power tools.

I change tactics with David. I tell him that my saying I am an MD has blocked many a conversation when I meet friends of friends at dinner parties; the subject of my work has to be avoided as something indecent on these occasions (if someone sick were present they would corner me later) although there is a genuine interest in medicine culturally, almost an overeagerness to hear the details. As with sex-talk, there is a mysteriousness wrapped around a center of condemnation.

I go on and on to David, unspooling opinions about the country and doctors as a group and me in particular and back again, ending with, "It's a vertical profession, this business I'm in. Like a telephone pole with spikes coming out which makes the pole look as if it has been stabbed, like it has a problem, but actually these spikes are critical for utility workers like me who are willing to climb."

"Nice metaphor," he says. "But here's the problem with all your blithering. It is not a vertical profession. It's horizontal. Your patients are horizontal and your work is lateral work."

●

When it is time to examine Mr. Dittus, I think of this conversation with David. The physical exam follows the history-taking, when doctor and patient have come to know each other a bit and there is a mutual understanding that diagnosis involves some frisking of the disease in the body on the bed. The lateral work, as David put it.

"The disease in the body on the bed"; such a phrase suggests that I am a cold man. Perhaps it makes me sound cruel and cheerfully enthusiastic. What I am trying to do is honestly represent the effect of repetition on my spirit. When a doctor sees a patient sitting or lying in a hospital room they think first: what disease? What happened? They do not think: father of two, nature lover, airplane pilot, I wonder if she enjoys cantatas?

When I first met Liz, she and I got into a conversation about using canned speeches with patients. She quickly gave me an example from her pediatric ophthalmology practice that very day. It was the way she spoke to the parents of a child whom she had just operated on. "I'm looking forward to seeing you again soon. But you have to get little Jimmy to wear the patch. They have to wear the patch every day. I know you are a responsible parent. Making them wear the patch, even when they don't want to, is like making them wear seatbelts. I know you make them wear seatbelts, because I know you're responsible." Et cetera. She said this several times each day; she could do it without thinking. She said it because she knew the effect it would have on the parent, and the effect on how that parent thought of her. I told her I had similar verbal patterns spinning in my head, the same verbal placebos.

We both felt bad about it and agreed that we truly did want patients to do well; in general, Liz and I liked our patients. Why couldn't we, then, free ourselves from this nonsense talk at a time of such great and often tragic importance to our patients? The disproportion in meaning between us and our patients while giving these speeches made us feel worse. Wasn't it pathetic that our patter was the same as a ballpark frank-peddler's: Dogs here! Get your dogs! Our patients' true gratitude had become only minimally gratifying to us.

Liz and I went into this depressing but mutually supportive spiral, a spiral that was itself most gratifying, until David interrupted us with pipe-smoke.

"Yes. Pygmies are amazed by mirrors," David said. "But that doesn't mean that mirrors aren't amazing."

The lateral work of patient examination begins just after I say my usual to George: "Why don't you take off your clothes and I'll be right back to examine you."

While this request begins with a questioning word (why) that usually allows the possibility of denial, I have spoken no question mark at the end and mean there to be none when I offer these words. Yet I am always amazed at the yielding. Certain words have great power and I think of this sentence as one of those extraordinarily well-understood, muscular word packages. I would include in this collection, "Stop or I'll shoot," and "Open the door, it's the police." Sumo-phrases, difficult to refuse. In *The Unbearable Lightness of Being*, Milan Kundera's womanizing doctor takes his medical training out of the hospital and as part of foreplay says simply, "Strip." I have always admired this coming directly to the point, and this shortening of the terms of my examination question would save me time on the wards (and imply the efficiency that often follows) and has probably been used for this effect during army pre-induction physicals for years. So far, I have avoided this abbreviation during my ward duties.

As I am parting the curtains to let myself out of Mr. Dittus's space so that he can have some privacy, I say over my shoulder "You can leave on your shorts." This add-on always has two effects. First, it makes those persons who aren't wearing underwear—and a surprising number of people never do (a fact that, as a medical student, confused me far more than the incidence of any disease I learned about)—suddenly feel embarassed. For some, this presumption on the part of their doctor only confirms that doctors are strangers and know nothing about the home's essential habits. The second effect is that they realize the doctor who just asked a seemingly innocuous "clothes-off" question has made clear their medical power by the more specific follow-up direction: keep or discard certain coverings.

I wait just outside the curtain, studying the three others who share Mr. Dittus's room and the room itself. The beds are arranged two and two. Mr. Dittus's A-bed is the first on the left as you come in, and as you move clockwise it goes B, C, D, with a wall of windows between B and C that is straight ahead. The windows are glass but have a plastic rainbowing sheen to them; they never look clean compared to the white of the sheets. They have small openings at the bottom to let in wind and the noise of the highway 100 yards off that runs parallel to the river. Two movie screen shades can be pulled down, each blocking half the room's light. The walls are off-white, giving the place its dimness. Each bed has a brown nightstand next to it that looks to be made of paneling, as well as a handy brown levitating breakfast tray contraption that slides up and down like the duck-ruler I keep in the foyer at home to measure my growing children. Each bed also has side-bars that can be arranged in a cage-effect. Skinny silver poles hold clear intravenous fluid bags (they remind me of the bags in which I brought goldfish home from the fish store when I was a child) that lead to the arms of the patients. Sympathy cards hang from the walls like dumb lips. Dishes of flowers sit along the ledge at the base of the window.

Two old men fill beds B and D. Every time I come to see Mr. Dittus they sit on their bed corners, cronies, hospital gowns falling away from their knees, men gone small with disease spitting their thick stuff into purple kidney bowls cleared once a shift by the nurses. These two gents keep their call buttons clasped to their gowns at lapel level where they look like mikes worn by talk show hosts. Bed C, diagonally across from Mr. Dittus, is taken by a guy around twenty years old who mostly keeps the sheet over his head so that all you can see is his seaweed hair poking out.

Mr. Dittus owns no underwear. He is stripped and relaxed when I reenter the curtains. He has a way of holding still to be looked at, like a foreign leader in state. I remember my father telling me about enlisting for World War II, describing the scene of thousands of men standing democratically naked in line for their first inspection. I imagine one never forgets the unease of that nakedness at the end of adolescence, at the beginning of war, which makes all future medical examinations seem inconsequential.

I have never figured out the proper approach to a naked patient lying prone. If they greet you sitting up they make it clear that they are going to keep at least a semblance of free will in all that follows. Greek medical manuals, according to Herodotus, declared a certain posture as the appropriate one for a doctor examining a patient. "When seated, his feet should be in a vertical line straight up as regards the knees, and be brought together with a slight interval. Knees a little higher than the groins and the interval between them such as may support and leave room for the elbows." I often wished it were so clear to me, but no doctor ever examined a patient while sitting since the Greeks.

Mr. Dittus has his hands behind his head and his ankles crossed. I draw the sheet up between his legs to his waist (a white fig leaf) and sit him up, starting at the top, getting a good look at those ears. Only a few parts of the exam generally matter and there is little scientific evidence offering any good reason for the "complete annual physical" that has been mythically recommended. A blood pressure reading, a going over of the skin, perhaps a well-placed, probing finger are all probably worthwhile if the goal is to pick up problems at a point when we can do something to save lives. Although it is apocalyptic so to say, the remainder of the exam is done to make the patient feel they are getting their money's worth. Generally, it is time-consuming and fruitless.

Mr. Dittus's skin is dry and my hand is dry. I feel the pulses in his neck and remember that before the unit of the second was invented, people used to time short events by their pulses. A corner-cutter, I focus on his complaint of chest pain which leads me to his heart.

The heart was the first organ my son talked about during kindergarten. I remember him to this day, soft-lipped and blue-eyed, big knees popping out of his shorts, saying, "The heart pumps blood to your body." I had to agree. "But the teachers say it doesn't pump blood to your brain," to which I raised an eyebrow but said nothing, giving his teachers the benefit of the doubt. "Celery is healthy food," my son also told me.

The heart is a trickier place to reach when examining a woman. When I say to a woman patient, "Why don't you take off your clothes and I'll be right back to examine you," staggeringly complex and subtle things happen that are hidden beneath cordiality. Doctors' fingers are filled with pity and desire; both lead to a certain kind of touching; neither patient nor doctor can tell which is the foremost emotion.

Not long ago a colleague of mine wrote an essay about his days as an intern twenty years before and his attraction to a brave young woman patient dying of cancer. His essay included the lines: "she was quite pretty," "I know I was attracted to her," "I passed her room perhaps eleven or twelve at night and saw that she was up . . . This time I was aware of some sexual tension in our conversation," "I remember that when she made the statement that doctors don't pay attention to your real needs, it felt like an invitation."

"I don't care what happened," his wife said to him when she read the essay. "You sound like a pervert."

She was a lawyer and convinced that if he were ever sued by a woman, these essays would be used against him in court.

Which recalls those matrons who in the early years of this century covered the legs of pianos and chairs with cloth supposing that, if they were left uncovered, the minds of men would wander from piano legs to human legs.

My colleague's essay always makes me wonder. Perhaps I should not see female patients. There are certainly women who refuse to see male doctors after bad experiences or from fear of lechery. These days a woman who chooses a male doctor is at best a naif. On the other side is my mother-in-law, always the contradictor, who thought it was "ridiculous" that her seventy-year-old male doctor even bothered to re-cover her breasts—he used paper towels which seemed odd to me—after he had examined them. Although choice is always preferred in America, perhaps male patients should only see male doctors and female patients, female doctors. There should be no collaboration with the enemy.

Unlike George Dittus, women always cover as much as possible when I walk in. To get to the heart, the left side of the gown has to be lowered, the left breast trespassed (or as surgeons write in their martial phrase, "mobilized") as the stethoscope is positioned. Women doctors I know and admire sometimes have had the same troubling hesitancies examining penises and testicles and have a tendency to avoid this part of the check-up. In medical school, my classmates and I had been taught the pelvic exam by "live models." These women, almost all of whom had had abusive experiences in this realm with doctors, were convinced that reparation was preferable to revenge and had decided to educate the next generation, us. About ten of us students gathered and learned from them as they allowed themselves to be serially examined, explaining to us what should be said as well as done, and the difficulties and discomforts involved. They were minimally paid by the medical school, but not one of them revealed what had happened that lead them to participate in this bizarre but incredibly educational exercise. I could never imagine men volunteering in this way with their bodies.

Years later, I still admit that I will never understand women's bodies in the rivalrous, and therefore more complete, way that I know men's.

•

Concern about the health of my own heart began soon after my father died. At thirteen, this vigilance took the form of avoiding anything sweet. I had come to believe that sweet foods caused heart disease. Not because my father ate sweets or was overweight. It was just something I decided.

I avoided candy, cakes, all soda, gum, cookies. When my friends' parents asked why I wasn't having dessert, I lied. "I don't like dessert," I told everyone. They told me they'd never heard of a child not liking dessert, but they made their own kids cut back, figuring I had some special knowledge that hadn't been made public yet.

I kept up this diet through high school. On my first date in college I passed on the ice cream after my burger and fries. My date, a decisive girl, loved ice cream and she sat there eating it alone. I never saw her again.

With my next date, when I refused to share a Carvel, I decided to explain myself. I never saw her again either.

My mother figured it out when I was fifteen. She asked, "Are you worried about your health?"

"Not much," I told her. But she knew lying. She told me that sweets had nothing to do with heart disease, but I didn't believe her either.

•

My stethescope is barely down.

"I've got to get home. It sounds fine in there, I'm sure. Let's celebrate," Mr. Dittus says.

Up to this point, he has been silent. I believed he wasn't concentrating on what I was doing.

I listen and hear nothing wrong. The heart produces its two rolling-through-a-footstep sounds, the sounds on either side of the arch, over and over again. I finish my exam quickly: the rest of his body is like a pumpkin three weeks after Halloween, soft, flabby. He reminds me of my father.

Before he speaks, George makes a humming sound, I believe out of nervousness or deference although I realize it may be just habit. "My foot is what hurts," he says, but I ignore him. His heart is the primary problem (whether he admits it or not) until the blood tests return telling us whether there has been any heart muscle injury, a heart attack. Chest pain will be virtually the only problem I consider when I draw my five-by-eight index card of George Dittus out of my pocket.

I say, "It does sound good in there. We'll wait a day for the blood test results." I am standing over his right side, this naked man.

He says, "*You* wait. I'm ready to go home." He looks at me with pity. I realize he is the sort who goes out to eat dinner every night and to just one place, a place that has mismatched chairs and a television that stays on all day and night. A man of ritual. I imagine him as sad, but this is probably wrong. I judge that he isn't going to leave without permission.

I say, "Relax. Take a day off. "

He nods his head so slowly as I speak that I doubt the truth or seriousness of what I am saying.

"I'm going to get dressed," he says. "You know why I listen to you? Because I look ridiculous."

•

I need to get back to the examination of women by men for one moment for I would forfeit my claim on truthfulness if I didn't admit here my memory of one woman patient I found attractive. I was a twenty-three-year-old medical student in New York City and a young woman who had been accidentally kicked in the stomach the night before during a fight at a dance club was admitted with severe abdominal pain. The senior doctors were concerned that she was at risk for bleeding internally. I was assigned the task of examining her abdomen regularly to make sure it remained soft.

When I say I was assigned this exam, I should say I assigned myself although it was a reasonable thing to do and I cleared it with my seniors (all men); she *was* admitted for close observation. I remember she had a deep tan and I ventured only between her ribs and her navel every three hours until 11:00 PM when she asked me to relent so she could sleep. I never looked her in the eye but her abdomen did remain soft during my look-out.

This is sordid and pathetic and I can imagine no woman doctor admitting to such repetitive excursions. But if I cannot tell about myself as a patient, then I must tell about myself as an examiner. In sympathy with my essay-confessing colleague, I must report this episode, however misconceived. His misdeed was only in his heart and seems trivial compared to my impropriety. But the reaction to his essay speaks to a great and pervasive concern about intimacy among doctors and patients, a concern that does not allow easy explanations. In this way, discussions of doctor-patient improprieties are like discussions of scientific fraud, where the marginal and half-conscious case is more interesting than the overt case, which is rare.

As I write about that disco-battered, over-examined midsection I am reminded of once stopping to use a phone at a stranger's house when my VW broke down. I remember the controlling way she stood at the door in her pants suit checking that I went to the phone and no where else. The alertness in her eyes said I was not to stray. With most patients it is this way too.

•

I write my note in Mr. Dittus's chart immediately after examining him. A quick note means I am up-to-date, have considered his care and have stated my opinions. If something goes wrong, it is not my fault.

The patients' charts are kept on a rollable stand beside the unit secretary's desk. Each chart is a small binder that a coach might use to keep a record of fastest times. Even today, when truth-telling is a mania, the custom of closed records remains, I suppose from a belief that the material therein is not suitable for the ill sensibility. Patients do not see their charts unless they expressly ask for them and I have watched a genuine confusion ensue as to what the proper response to this unusual request is, as if there were a Lee Harvey Oswaldian uncertainty. (The certain answer here, in a profession of real and consistent uncertainties, is to turn over the goods).

I remember reading that the medical case history began in its current form around the time of Poe (although Poe was interested in and publicized the orderly detective-hunt of the medical note, his genius was most aroused by the autopsy). Written according to strict rules and structured around the organ systems, the chart note now reports the history taken from the patient, (emplotment the litcrits call this section, although that is clearly too cemetaryesque a term), followed by the physical exam, the results of blood tests, X-rays, urine analyses, and electrocardiograms. In the case of Mr. Dittus, as in the cases of the fourteen other patients on my ward, I include what happened (chest pain) as well as what didn't happen (he didn't lose his breath) but which might nonetheless pertain. I include not one answer to the questions I might have been interested in asking (but don't ask), questions that might be important in the days that follow: What do you *think* happened to you? How do you bear adversity? How long do you expect to live? In this four-bed room, over what do you have power? What if you lost this power? What was the worst pain you have ever experienced? What was the worst suffering? Were these the same? What if that suffering had not been relieved?

I don't ask any of these questions because I don't want to know the answers. They are too dangerous; they are what persons in love might talk about, not doctor and patient. If, as Rilke said, love requires a "shortening of the senses," doctoring should be love's opposite. In training, I was taught to want none of love's blur. Although I was to work close-in, I would want to avoid this danger, I learned.

While my patients begin as solids, as persons, men and women, they become concepts as I write in their charts: the flesh made word. I write none of the things I actually know about Mr. Dittus: that he is restless and slightly disconnected, that he is incapable of pretense, that his heart disease (he had had a heart attack two weeks before, I learn from reading the previous notes in an old chart—his medical record—which arrives from storage in the basement) is a great mystery to him, that his opinions are emphatic and simpleminded. In short, that he is one weird number, and has roughed up the memory of my father.

I write short notes. After speaking with a patient, writing it down always feels imprecise and unengaging. Also I have a particular view of the chart note. My notes are meant to prejudice and intimidate as well as provide the simple facts. This is the very opposite of literature. Now it's true that literature often takes off from true incidents, case reports: Flaubert drew *Madame Bovary* from a newspaper account (Julian Barnes discusses this) and *Lord Jim* replicated an 1880 London Times account of the S.S. Jeddah—the single case, artfully rearranged can have great power. But literature is meant to engross using conjecture and outrageousness, while medical notes are simply mental shorthand. Psychiatrists (and their cousins the neurologists, like Oliver Sacks, whose notes I imagine are sweaty and illegible) write longer notes, symptom stories. They mean their long notes to be individual while my internist notes are trying to be like every other internist note. There is no invention in my notes; they are chilly. There is nothing unanticipated (again the opposite of art) because I follow a pattern. What I write is immeasurably shallow but the absence of complexity brings great joy to my readers, other doctors, who appreciate that I can take a patient's life and bring it in under a page. Simple and straightforward, it seems honest (sometimes I write in a full exam even if I haven't checked the eyes, all the reflexes). If a true writer is one who can make a riddle out of an answer, a doctor is the opposite.

In my final assessment, I write that the chest pain Mr. Dittus described might be (1) another heart attack, one portion of the heart muscle suffering irreversible injury due to a completely blocked coronary artery that fed the muscle blood with oxygen (it never makes sense to my wife, why the heart, which pumps blood, which bathes in blood, needs to have blood specially fed to it), or (2) angina (the heart muscle temporarily deprived of blood, but recovering, screaming out in pain), or (3) some pain having nothing to do with the heart. I write that number two is the most likely possibility. I write that he has high blood pressure that may be playing a part and needs to be controlled, here, now. I include nothing about the pain in the foot that Mr. Dittus has complained about. I have no explanation for his foot pain and therefore it is not worthy of comment. (This same trick in a marriage eventually leads to divorce.) I mean to prejudice and intimidate in order to leave no doubts about the action that needs to be taken in the treatment of Mr. Dittus.

I am an omniscient narrator as I follow the time-honored system of the chart. I am so omniscient I allow no one else to speak in my note, not Mr. Dittus or his nurse; there are no quotations from my patients. I have seen patient quotations in the notes of other doctors, but these inclusions only call out for explanations. There must be no mysteries. The zealousness of my notes please me. Meanwhile, my overriding emotion is: I hope I don't miss anything.

•

I have made it seem as if my written evaluation of Mr. Dittus makes up the entire width of his chart. This is not the case. If, at the end of a patient's stay, you took up their chart and went through it page by page you will find, actually, many pages of detail. The very first page is a review of basic facts—patient name, date of birth, home address, next-of-kin, insurance status, religion—the facts on my five-by-eight card.

The next page is a Patient Personal Property Information Sheet. Here, there is a list of what the patient places in the hospital safe deposit box. (I'm not sure where this safe is located in our hospital.) There is a checklist: cash, bank book, credit cards, ID cards, keys, personal papers, rings, wallet, walkers/canes/crutches/ braces, watch, glasses, jewelry, hearing aid, dentures. The essentials.

The third page comes from the emergency room listing all that happens when first examined and while waiting on a stretcher in that cold, drafty place. Then comes a section of the Progress Notes, as I have described, with doctors recording their daily evaluations. Then thick, carbon-copy pages called PHYSICIAN ORDERS, where the medications, oxygen, blood tests, et cetera, that the patient is to have are written. In small print on the bottom of these order pages is the advice: medication orders must be written in the metric system only. This advice is ignored and suggests that the company that produces these pages is based overseas. Following the ORDERS section are laboratory results.

Why in 1999, at the edge of the millenium, when all this information can be put directly into a computer, we need any of these papers is beyond me.

After all of this essential information, near the end, are the Nursing Sheets. These are pages with boxes to be checked, dividing the patient's history and examination into yes/no possibilities. Was this patient short of breath? Does this patient have jaundice? Does this patient have leg swelling? The same information that the doctor should have recorded in the progress note but here in a standardized format. The implication of this doctor-nurse disparity is that nurses can't be trusted to record free-hand; they need boxes to be complete. These pages are last because doctors never look back there. Who cares what nurses think? is the logic, I presume. Of course the nursing notes contain essential information that can be found nowhere else: specific patient goals, patient's family and home situation, pattern of sleep, personal habits, ability to care for themselves. Notes from social workers, physical therapists and other non-doctors are lumped into the nursing notes.

Nursing care is traditionally disrespected by doctors. In the cafeteria, I hear it: nurses are women who agree to exploitation; nurses' care produces nothing tangible while cardiologists open arteries, and surgeons bypass tumors; nurses are "stewardesses on a very clean plane."

All this seems strange to me. The health professions are sometimes called the caring professions and from any reasonable viewpoint, the nurses are the most caring. But there is something about nursing care that makes doctors anxious. In my younger days I thought it was the emotion involved in their work, the sentimentality. Later I realized that their minute-to-minute, hands-on work had led me to the false belief that nurses were coddlers, and coddlers were morally suspect. More recently I realized that nurses are simply more willing to have meaningful moments with patients than I am.

I have never rubbed ointment onto a patient's body. I have never squeezed in onto a patient's back and rubbed it into the flesh where I thought pain was coming from while their eyes were closed. I believe that I have helped patients and I have sensed pain and touched it, but I have never achieved this intimacy in my medical life. I have never touched in simple and comforting motions their bodies, which are their medical histories. I have never made their skin red and healthy, if only for a moment, with the heat of my hands.

•

On Tuesday morning, my *Medicine World News* is sitting on top of my desk when I arrive at 8:00 AM. The bulk of the mail comes in around 11:30, but this newspaper gets there early and my secretary leaves it on top of an uneven pile of articles that I have torn from medical journals but have not yet found time to read. I mean to read them in order to improve myself as well as protect myself against the energetic ambition of my students who I'm sure regret having to correct my unfamiliarity with the cutting edge. My secretary sorts my mail. Her name is Marie. She is ten years older than I am, has two boys in high school, worries about her health insurance payments, and regularly tells me that she has more life experience than I have. I find it hard to believe that I have a secretary most days.

At home, I start off *The New York Times* with the headlines, followed by the book review, the business pages, and the editorials; I finish with the tasty B-section, the disasters. During my months on the wards, I also read the obituaries in our local paper while my wife, in dashes of blue ink, finishes the *Times* puzzle with a conquering smile. Obituaries are written in some universal language at some undefined grade school level so that our local paper's read like the *Times'*. Except for the pictures. Our paper includes photos of the deceased and although I find these images next to the text disconcerting, they're also fascinating. My wife won't look; who wants to see them, still alive, hair combed flat, smiling like it isn't so bad, she asks. I read the obituaries simply to find out if one of my patients has died during the evening before without my having heard. My ward team does not usually wake me with death calls if I know the patient was about to die, or if the patient or their family has made clear that they desire no further treatment. But as the senior doctor ultimately and legally responsible, I always want to know about unexpected deaths. Sometimes, however, my team doesn't call when they should, so I read the obituaries looking for names I know.

No, that's not true: I read the obituaries to see if I have been blamed for a death, my name squeezed in just after "long illness" and "died in the hospital" and before the names of the loved ones.

At work, with my *Medicine World News*, I always open first to the section "Medicolegal Decisions" that begins around page 32. These reports usually run for about three pages with bold headers such as PHYSICIAN PRE-SCRIBES, COURT CONVICTS followed by six or seven paragraphs of text that snake around three-color pharma-ceutical ads and describe the nation's interesting medicine-related malpractice cases, the physician's defense, and the courts' findings. There are about ten cases listed in each weekly issue. I read these legal notes with my feet kicked up on my desk balancing with that about-to-tip thrill and with the feeling that all of American medicine is capsizing. It is obvious: around the country, the public is mad, has gone mad.

This reading used to bring me pleasure. The angry tone of the plaintiffs sings out; it is a harmony I recognize. There are several types of cases. There are the unsurprising, dis-couraging, mildly humorous cases against individual doc-tors: PATIENT HAS HERNIA ON LEFT, SURGERY ON RIGHT, or BURNED BY LAMP IN OPERATING ROOM, where the surgeon, rather than bringing over another lamp in order to get better light into the operative area, removed a protective lens from a light and repositioned it nearer to the patient's foot, severely burning it. Next, there are the sickening cases against hospitals: a mother without health insurance brings in her thirteen-year-old daughter with stomach pains and is told no one will see her unless she makes a $50 payment which she can not do. She leaves without treatment and the daughter's appendix bursts hours later. There are the suspect doctor stories: PHYSICIAN DENIED DEA CERTIFICATE, the certificate needed to dispense controlled substances, because he purchased twenty ounces of pharmaceutical-grade cocaine for "office use" during a twenty month period. Other plastic surgeons testified that use of one ounce of cocaine per month was excessive. Except (surprise!) if he was addicted. There are the novelistic, ironic cases, the ones you couldn't make up: a doctor who is on trial for leaving a drain in the leg of a patient for months after surgery, another who administers aid to a juror who suffers a heart attack during a recess. These events are "so extraordinarily prejudicial" a mistrial is required.

At dinner parties, I'm often told local versions of these bad doctor tales. I hear all the bad stories, the lawsuits-to-be, and so as not to be a disagreeable guest, rather than defending the whole profession, I always agree with the complaints. Sometimes, feeling playful, I even help with evidence against the doctors whom the main-course story is about. If the party is a bore, I offer some details from one of the court decisions I've read that week.

HUSBAND LIABLE FOR WIFE'S MEDICAL BILL is a party favorite. The patient's husband did not know his wife went to the hospital. She was an inpatient for fifteen days and was billed $9000. She paid $1500 and the hospital filed suit against the husband for the remainder of the bill. The economics of the suit usually leads to a discussion, with silverware banging aggressively, about this marriage in particular and then marriages in general. We move on to escalating loyalty claims ("I couldn't stand if my spouse was gone for even one day"), and the subject of spouses spending time apart leads naturally to extramarital affairs, and who we at the table know (and aren't at the table) who might be having an affair, and by then everyone is thinking of themselves in a more critical but self-satisfied way hoping for dessert to arrive. During coffee, I often tell those at the table that the Missouri court had required the husband to pay his wife's medical expenses and we start all over again, cream sloshing in gesturing hands: husband against wife, husbands against wives, with the occasional brave soul crossing gender lines as we retire to the living room.

It used to be that the medicolegal notes not only brought me pleasure, they made me giddy. For a few reasons. First, because I have not yet been sued and therefore can think to myself, "Nyah, Nyah" as I read. Although at its root this response is actually a form of gratitude, it has attached a feeling of superiority. Not having been sued is a judgement in favor of my abilities. This gulp of superiority sometimes leaves a bad aftertaste coming as it does at the expense of patient suffering in these cases, but it also allows for a certain self-confidence that is necessary to keep intact in order to do my work. All years of training beyond the first few, I have always believed, are a matter of confidence and speed: what took three hours and three facts previously, later takes one minute and one clinical fact. Speed grows out of confidence. But my giddiness also springs from a superstitious fear. I believe that some elusive knowledge can be gathered from these rulings if I read carefully enough, and this will protect me from the inevitable instance when I appear in "Medicolegal Decisions," which might not be so far off.

When I write in a medical chart, I write quickly and confidently. And as I write I often think: Why must I be childishly right with each patient assessment? And the answer is: *So I do not show up in medicolegal Notes.* This single fear, present in the write-up of every single case, instructs my unyielding, pseudo-factual note-style. At the end of each note, I also cleverly exaggerate my already illegible penmanship into two gashes that are meant to represent my name and make it disappear at the same time, another magical-thinking way of protecting myself from the inevitable lawsuit. But you can always make out the MD.

•

There is so much I don't know about my father. It's a family joke that whenever we get together at an anniversary or wedding or funeral, I go around and ask any older relative what they remember about my father. "Go away. You asked me this last time," they say. They are not amused at my persistence. I'm a grown man, but I can't stop. I get excited by the prospect of some new speck of information. And what else is there to talk about? Eastern Europe? Stocks? Hurricanes?

Memories of my father are all good. One hundred percent. Perhaps this is because my bad-memory-line is clogged by Gresser. Perhaps I should be thankful for Gresser killing him, allowing the pure filtrate of pleasant memories. I think of Gresser as a large man, a clogger, a man of bulk and threat. Unattractive.

Does anyone who watches me during the day—my students, the nurses, my patients—see the combat that goes on in me, notice the moment that I am denouncing Gresser in my mind (this happens most often at work when the tools of medicine are apparent), insulting him, settling scores? No, of course not. But my wife sees. She knows I don't sleep well and when I wake her, she says in the dark, half-kidding, "I don't know you. What's your name again?"

•

As I am seeing another patient on 9A, Lynn comes up behind me.

"You better go see our friend Mr. Dittus," she says.

"Don't tell me. He wants to go home," I say.

"Not exactly," she says. "But close."

I resist the urge to say, "I'll come back and see him later," or "Call the intern or resident, they can take care of whatever it is and let me know if there's a problem," or simply, "I'm too busy to deal with him right now." Lynn wants me to go.

I walk down the hall, the fluorescent lights sizzling overhead. Lynn walks a step behind me, filling me in every few steps.

"He's been pacing all night . . . ."

"You know how he's supposed to be on bed rest. He wasn't . . . ."

"He says he wants to see the guy in charge . . . ."

Mr. Dittus is pacing in front of his bed, a guard dog, a few steps forward, a pivot, then back again with his little limp. When he sees me, he points diagonally across the room to Bed C and says, "That man's a junkie and I want to get out of this room."

I look across and see a young black man, perhaps thirty-five years old, the man who had been under his sheets every other time I visited the room, laying on top of his sheets with a pained expression.

"How could you put me in a room with a junkie? Aren't there special places for them? How could you put any of us with him?"

The other two men in the room are silently staring at us.

"Calm down, Mr. Dittus," Lynn says.

"I will not! He's a junkie, know what I mean? You're a good man. Do something."

"George, what makes you think that," Lynn says. I am glad to see that she isn't having much success with Mr. Dittus either.

"Listen," he says to me. "Is he your patient too?"

"No," I say.

"Look, I want some control over this," George says.

"Has he been bothering you?" I ask.

"I can't sleep here, with him here."

"Has something happened?" I ask. Usually, the longer a patient is in the hospital, the less I think about them. Certainly the most acute thinking occurs on the day they arrive, as I write the first note. When a new problem arises, it means taking a history all over again.

"He's an addict. He's an addict. What other possibility is there? Look at his feet."

The man's feet look fine. Pink-soled, black man's feet like the inside of a mouth. He has a thick gold chain around his neck.

"Did he do anything we should know about?" I feel like the police.

"An animal," George mumbles. "Just an animal." Then he says louder, "I don't know what kind of game you're trying to play here, but it's simple. Move me out of here. That's all I'm saying."

I don't want to hear any more of this. I am anxious to get outside. This isn't my job.

"Or send me home," George says.

"All right, new room," I say.

"Now we're getting somewhere."

George goes over to his wardrobe unit, a locker next to the sink, and takes out his coat and puts it on. He is wearing those spongy slippers, one-quarter inch green foam, and he looks silly with a windbreaker over a hospital gown.

"A semi-private is fine," George says.

I think (in the middle of all this): what an absurd term: semi-private. Places are either private or not private. But I know what he means and I know our hospital has no two-person rooms in this building, only singles and four-beds and we try to save the singles for those with contagious diseases like tuberculosis, and for maniacs, like those waking up after an overdose.

Lynn nudges me and I go up to the man in bed C who still watches us calmly.

"How you doing?" I ask, trying to play it cool. But I don't know what to say to him and I make several false starts, "I'm not sure . . . . There's been a lot of confusion . . . ." Then I say, "Anyway, you'll have a new roommate soon enough." Before I turn away, I try to get a good look at him, to see if I believe that he is an addict.

Not that you can always tell such things simply by looking at an overburdened man's face. But I have an intuition about addicts because running this ward team I have cared for my share of them and one look is sometimes good enough. Also I have recently lived across the street from an addict. I didn't know it when we bought the house. Our realtor told us the rumor but we didn't believe her and we had seen the house on three sunny days. The neighborhood seemed fine. Now I know: always shop for houses at night.

Leaving George's room, and returning to the low-ceilinged, uncomfortably air-conditioned hall, I ask Lynn, "Do you think that guy's a drug abuser?"

"Drug *user*," she correct me. "Abuser is too judgmental."

"Right. Do you?" I know she has everyone in the room as her patient.

"As a matter of fact, I know most definitely that he is not a drug user," she says.

"He took it all pretty well," I say.

"He doesn't speak a word of English," she says. "He's actually from French Guinea. He arrived in a plane a week ago and it turns out he has lung cancer."

"That young guy has lung cancer? No wonder he looks so bad. How did he end up here?"

"His sister actually lives here, believe it or not. And when she first came in with all this gold on, you'll be glad to know that everyone treated the two of them like drug addicts. It turns out that his father is Guinea's ambassador to France and they're all from the royal family. He came to the United States for treatment."

"I see," is all I could say.

"And he got a four-bedder because he didn't know to ask for anything else," she says.

We start walking back toward the nurse's station so I can finish writing my notes and Lynn can begin the arrangements for getting George a private room.

•

Before seeing any patients, I meet with my team of interns, residents, and medical students to hear the events of the last day and to make plans for the upcoming days. There has been a lot of patient turnover; a young man with an intolerable headache and a woman bleeding from her stomach have gone home, and several new people have arrived on our ward. I learn that among our fifteen patients we now have four whose last name is Johnson, one who has just arrived from a nursing home with a bloodstream infection and is about to die. We are caring for a lawyer, an exotic male dancer and a jewelry carder. We have a woman trucker who broke down bodily on one of our state's fine highways, and a laundress with a stroke. The rest of our new ones are between jobs or unemployed and their bodies have become undependable.

My favorite is an eighty-three-year-old man with abdominal pain. He came to the emergency room with his wife, and when it was decided that he would have to stay overnight in the hospital, she refused to leave him. So she was admitted to the hospital as well; she was dehydrated in sympathy with his inability to eat, but mostly her willpower led to the admission. The two were settled in different rooms. I hear this touching story from Mr. Viera's nurse before I go to see him. During my interview with him he tells me he's glad to be in a room different from his wife's. In fact, he wouldn't mind if I could send him to a nursing home for a few weeks away from her so he can get a rest. "She complains too much," he tells me. "She won't leave me alone. Help me doctor, please."

•

I hear the update on George Dittus, who should have slept well, who should have been happy as could be in his new, private room. I am annoyed at George for creating extra work for me and the nurses (and for his false accusation of the young prince) but this annoyance disappears when the first thing I learn is that Mr. Dittus has indeed had a heart attack according to the blood tests we have been drawing over the past twenty four hours.

"Does he know?" I ask my team.

"We just got the results," my intern answers.

"He's not going to be happy. Mostly because he thinks he's geting out of here today and now he's going to have to stay awhile."

"Mr. Dittus had a little problem last night," my intern says.

"Again?" I ask.

"A different problem. He fell."

"What happened?" I ask.

"He just fell. Well, and he lacerated his forehead. He got four stitches."

"He passed out?" I ask, worried that his heart was acting up again, not pumping enough to his brain.

"Tripped," he says. "And he wants to see you."

I ride the elevator up to 9A from our conference room on 5A. It is stunningly slow and stops on every floor. They have changed the interior for the third time in a year, back to carpeting on the floors and walls. A coffin with a fan vent. When I come into Mr. Dittus's room he asks for the twentieth time, "Are you the one in charge?"

"Yes I am," I tell him.

He says, "Could you fix this band-aid on my head?"

A white gauze pad is dangling over his eye, half its adhesive gone, swinging back and forth like the look-out on a New York City apartment door.

"Bad fall," I say. "What happened?"

"I've been telling you guys for days about my foot. Nobody even looks at it. No one has looked at it yet. The damn thing's swollen. It hurts. I'm limping, if you hadn't noticed. I banged it and I tripped. I told the other guy this." He doesn't say it in a pleading way, and he's not looking for comfort.

I give him my easy-does-it, surface look of concern. "Let me check it for you."

He takes off his green foam hospital slipper and I kneel to look at his right foot. I'm not expecting to find a problem. His foot gives off the very faint smell of vinegar. Mr. Dittus's skin is as white as the stones sheep lick, marshmallow white. And there in the soft white flesh of the top of his right foot is one screaming red joint where the big toe attaches.

Gout.

Couldn't be anything else.

"Gout," I announce, keeping my voice flat like this was not unexpected. I'm not looking up at him and I end up screaming it. Actually, I'm stunned. Gout, I know, hurts like a hammer shot.

"You guys know a hell of a lot about nothing," he says. He's angry and I've never seen him angry. "Now fix this band-aid."

As I begin to replace his bandage, George says, "Don't you have a conscience?"

My face is close to his; his breath is strong and bitter.

"What do you mean?" I ask.

"I mean the shape my foot is in—look at the swelling."

"I'm sorry," I say. I can't remember the last time I said that to a patient.

I replace the bandage on his forehead, trying to keep my hands steady. I want to give George the hopeful news about his foot, that things will improve, but he is not interested in talking to me. I leave unnaturally, backing out.

After passing George's room three or four times while seeing other patients, I stop in.

"Medicine for my foot? Any ideas?" Mr Dittus asks. He looks relaxed. I realize that I haven't even seen him grimace. I have always had a jealous respect for people who tolerate pain. I am afraid to visit my dentist for a cleaning.

I hadn't mentioned a word about specific treatment during my last visit.

"I've taken care of it," I say. He might want the name of his pill-to-come. He might want to know about side effects, (they are actually just effects; the 'side' is meaningless if it happens to you). I rarely review medications in detail with patients unless they ask.

"A pill, I suppose," he says.

"Three times a day for a week or so, although your foot should feel better sooner than that."

"It's just gout," George says to me.

"Yeah."

"How does the medicine know to go just to my foot?" he asks me, but I don't know if he's kidding or if this is a serious question.

•

Although the TV image of a heart attack is someone wild-eyed and gasping, Mr. Dittus has already sailed past the big danger period with no further chest pain, no further symptoms whatsoever. His being sent to 9A from the emergency room had been bad judgement, but fortunately there had been no serious complications.

I am drawn to George Dittus, but I'm also suspicious of my attraction. It is so plainly a sign of unfinished struggle, of my weakness, of strange private remembrances of my father that should have been, by now, retired. Dittus is like the abrupt arrival of history, and he's shaken me loose from the habitual expectations of what a patient is.

When my team gave me the news that he had indeed suffered a heart attack, I had a flash of George as a dead man. At some point during the hospital stay of any patient, I think of what they would look like if they died. This thought led me to some practical questions. Who would come to identify George's body? Who would we notify? George repeatedly claimed that he had no living relatives.

One part of the day that nurses and doctors share is death, and dying is the image most people think of when they think of hospitals. Patients die around the clock on my ward with no preference for the day of the week, the roommate, the season, if it's sunny or rainy. If, as Nabokov wrote, fiction is gradually evolving to be more accurate about life, medicine is similarly evolving to be more accurate about death. We don't like to talk about any of this of course. I recently heard this joke: One man asks his friend, "Would you like to know the circumstances and the timing of your death?" And his friend answers, "No." And the first

71

man says, "Never mind then." That's just about the way we're all willing to discuss dying.

I am often asked by relatives of the dying about the circumstances and timing of the loved one's death. It's my job. I often try to soft-shoe it (that problem again of having to answer the same questions over and over) by reviewing the care we have given and so on, and I used to always end by saying something like, "death is a natural event." But no one believes me anymore. They expect death to take place in a hospital, and the more initials in the name of the place of death (ICU, CCU) the harder we doctors are trying. It's not a natural event at all anymore. At home, I call our hospital the White House in salute to the pale and dying.

I remember that the first dead person I ever saw was one I had to touch: my cadaver in medical school. Before anatomy, I had had no dread of seeing the dead. I had etherized frogs and even kept them cool in our refrigerator. If I found a bone in the woods, it interested me only if I imagined it was human. But by the end of that first semester of medical school, anatomy lab ("Lab" because it stunk, or because we wore white coats or because there was no blackboard or slide projector, and not because we did any experiments) had taken some of this empiricism out of me.

I remember the gagging smell of formaldehyde and the parts of her that looked human: the fingernails with polish, the pierced ears. I went home very upset that first day, lay on my bed and read Wallace Stevens, trying to use poetry as escape. And then I read this: "If her horny feet protrude, they come/ to show how cold she is, and dumb." I could not even depend on poetry to help me relax. The next day, I couldn't keep my eyes off her feet, but I had convinced myself that the rest of her might just have been wax. I didn't know why she gave her body to us or what she died from (there was a waiting list for the dead to get into our anatomy lab—folks finally nailing a spot in an Ivy league school), although we looked for causes as we dissected her.

I went to my first open-coffin wake soon after meeting my cadaver. By then I was reading about the dead incessantly. How cadavers were kept on ice until the late eighteenth century (except in ancient Egypt where they were salted.) How embalming began as a way of being able to keep people under glass containers, like pastries, or in natural bedroom settings where loved ones could come by and say hello. How, in funeral homes, dead eyes were smeared with vaseline to prevent drying and lids were closed two-thirds of the way for the appropriate look. How the corpse was "restored"; the dentures, glasses, cosmetics put in place. I had never been in a funeral home, just as I had never been in a police station, both of which were closer to my home than the supermarket, where I went at least once a week; these were places you went only if you had to. But once I appreciated how big a business death was—caskets, burial vaults, urns, headstones, monuments, hearses, dark-windowed limos—what a high-profit industry it was, I got more interested in my cadaver and her foresight in avoiding the huge price-tag.

During medical school, there was a belief among my non-medical friends that my working with a cadaver meant that I had some inside information about the dead. But this wasn't the case. I was glad when anatomy ended each day.

A different interest in the dead began only after I began to care for patients. The first time I got to know a person, tried to save them, failed, but at least helped them die, I will not forget. It was only then that I realized that anyone might have a fatal outcome, if not from disease, then from me, what I did or didn't do. I remember my first dead patient becoming an object so powerful that I needed to inspect him as I had inspected my cadaver years before. And inspect him in a way I had never inspected the living. I acted like my son, who, spying a dead sandshark on a beach, spent ten minutes circling. He walked around saying, "Can I touch it?" Then he'd lean over it, tiptoe around it, sit down next to it. Knowing something, he kicked sand on the dry-rotted creature.

My patient had died of leukemia. It was a drawn-out business that ended about 11:00 PM on a Saturday night with his brother on vigil down the hall in the waiting room. I walked the quiet corridor, pulled up a chair next to this sad, chunky man who I had seen virtually every day for a month and told him the news. He swung at me. A big, roundhouse right hand that I avoided by ducking my head between my knees. He started to tip off his chair with the effort and I pushed him back. That's when I smelled the bourbon. I stayed polite and told him to get back to me if he had other questions, and left him for the unit secretary to find with the paperwork. Then I walked back to my dead patient's room.

My patient had been a truly nice man, a florist who gave me orchids for my wife-to-be and whose room was a visual pleasure to visit; I was feeling real bad about the whole thing with his brother so I walked back to the room to check if he was truly dead (like my son kept doing as I tried to continue our walk down the beach), but by then the nurses were in with him. When they pulled back his covers and took his IV out, I stared at his penis, softish and swollen, its haughtiness gone.

Doctors never washed the corpse (or for that matter the live patient) like nurses did, and I watched but didn't join in. I didn't know what to do. They wrapped him in a morgue sheet, double wrapped him in fact, and lifted him, with my help, into a morgue cart that was sunken like a bathtub on wheels, sending him off to the basement where the pathologists did their steady work on the stalled bodies right next to Shipping and Receiving. Together, we checked his top drawer stuff—the ballpoint, the dimes, his cigars and flask (I suggested liquor for when the pain pills didn't kick in fast enough), a book of matches, his wallet and dentures.

In those first years of training I saw many dead folks. But after the first month or so of internship I had a predictable reaction different from sadness. Just after my patients died, I felt this primeval vigor, this anti-death energy. It took the form of potency; I thought about sex. All the sex/death connections the more embarassing writers offer (orgasm as in "impermanent eternal," you know the slop), is not what I'm speaking of here; I've never thought about death during sex. Only the opposite was true, I thought of sex during death. The body is where sex lives and I felt this dead person was giving their lust over to me. At the ends of others' lives, something woke in me. Some desire to stave off that waste, that the swindle was waiting for me too.

I didn't really feel good or bad about this; it seemed right; we are mortal, we just forget it sometimes and this was the opportunity to remember. The imagined antics that I could have been having with my wife usually lasted about five minutes and when I got on to other work was usually replaced by a giddiness that, in my thirties, regularly took an even more extreme form: Munchkin-speak. When I passed a fellow doctor who knew about my very sick, now-dead, patient, I would sing out: "She's not only merely dead, she's really most sincerely dead."

I don't expect George to die.

But he has now had two heart attacks in two weeks. Death is not out of the question at that rate.

•

If you spend your work-life expecting to get things right, expecting to figure them out fast, if you spend your life in pursuit like this, then you will probably have high expectations for everyone you come in contact with. I don't like gas lines, or supermarket check-out lines, or people who can't count change quickly, or bumper-to-bumper traffic. Because I expect this rightness (at least right thinking) of myself I don't often feel triumphant. I wish I did more often, but I don't. It's not like that, my work.

Still, it's a powerful secret to realize you know how these bodies work, or should work. In the evenings, sometimes, as I walk through the halls, what I hear is their bodies. I'm still learning the extent of my power. My wife used to say, "You're in love with it all, the white rooms, the patients, the helping. It isn't a job to you."

But what I tell her now is, "The New Medicine is coming. Yes it is."

Important men and women, administrators who have never had to look so neat in their cubbyhole lives, are getting their hair cut to go on TV and talk to the reporters about the changes that are coming. I turn on the news and most nights now I see a wave of them staring right at me talking about my medical future, talking mergers and operating margins. At the same time, a number of my medical friends are thinking of leaving their work. Leaving not in a blunt, adios sort of way, but just pulling back and disappearing. Surely the Haircut People know they will be forcing good people out, doctors who have their own personal reasons for quitting.

The Haircut People aren't afraid of me. Only my patients are afraid because they understand that I am responsible for their immediate world. This inevitably leads to fear, although one should never draw conclusions about the sick; you never know what to expect. The Haircut People are not sickly; they can't even imagine themselves among the sick. The sick wouldn't want the New Medicine, doctors sending in their hygienists like dentists do, then stopping by during the last ten seconds to probe once and ask about the wife. The sick won't want the New Medicine but they'll be too sick to say anything. That's the great advantage the Haircuts have.

At meetings, I've glimpsed their weekly reminder lists. The Haircut I sat next to last had written: Try to memorize the name of one employee each day. An admirable goal, but the compulsion to record this plan explained to me who this man was. Jolly and mean, he had an appetite for humiliation. In his briefcase were brochures for an executive pension plan and a tanning salon.

As for us doctors, the Haircut People figure that any group that's so dissatisfied with its work (polls, polls) must have done something awful and feels bad for itself anyway. Maybe we won't notice their bad decisions, at least until the uproar starts.

I'm not interested in competing in the arena of personal shame. And if I leave, I want to initiate my leaving.

When my best friend first told me of his plans for premature retirement about three months ago, I said simply, "Nah!" But now I listen more carefully, giving advice when unrequested, which I complain he does to me, and which, in retaliation, I have decided to do back.

This may all be mid-life stuff, I tell him. But later I think about it this way: if he wants to change his life, why shouldn't he give his energy to those who *aren't* dying?

•

I never saw my father dead.

I heard rasping across the hall from my room at 2:00 AM one September morning. I woke up and made my bed like I was late for school although it was still dark outside. I remember my windows were shut tight because there had been a chill that evening. I heard the doorbell ring and when I looked out my window, the red ambulance lights gyroscoped across my front lawn. All the other houses on the street were dark and the circling red lights bounced off every window. The ambulance was running; white smoke came from its tailpipe.

My mother let the ambulance men in, and when I heard them coming up the stairs I opened my door a crack. I knew it was my father (he'd been sick for months) they'd come for and I shut my door. I sat on my bed and looked out the window. I heard the scrape of metal out in the hall and men grunting as they lifted. When my mother knocked and told me to get ready to go to the hospital, my father was already in the ambulance.

We drove behind the ambulance the whole way. My eyes were closed. I wouldn't look at the back door of the ambulance, behind which I knew my father lay. They took him inside the hospital while my mother parked the car and then we went inside and sat in the molded chairs of a waiting room.

My mother left to see my father several times over the next hour but I did not.

He died at 4:15 AM and I refused to see him.

•

Tuesday afternoon and no one has yet given George the news about his heart attack. Who would have given it to him? I asked each member of my team if they would like to talk with George when they gave me the results of his blood tests at our morning conference. These interns and residents, housestaff they are sometime called, sit right in the middle of medicine's tradition of obedience, its absence of democracy. Interns and residents are in understandably awkward positions. They do important but numbing work (fill out papers, order tests, draw blood, retrieve lab results, call consultants, deal with nurses from minute to minute), while trying to steal time to read and learn, or go home to get reacquainted with their friends, children, beds. They want to please me, but there are parts of their work they don't mind avoiding (so they have time for other things) or having me do. Like Dukes and Duchesses, they need to be adaptable within the confines of class. I could have ordered one of them to speak with George. It is possible that one of them might have been tight with him and would have been willing to give him the news, but this wasn't the case: they wanted me to do the deed.

They are not ultimately responsible for decisions or outcomes. I am.

So I again return to 9A. I am visiting George quite often and I'm beginning to find his mustard yellow chair pretty comfortable.

Lynn is on duty. She stops me on the way in to see him. She says, "So George has gout, huh?"

"Yes he does." I'm waiting for her to humiliate me. She has the chance.

"How did the old boy take it? His temper is pretty obvious."

"Better than I did. You know, most people I see in my office once a year. I hear what they've been up to, about their kids, about their aches. I don't worry about them between visits. Seeing these people day after day is differ-

78

ent. I'm supposed to be thinking about them all the time. And then I miss his foot."

"I missed it too, you know. He wouldn't take his shoe off. Now, when I ask him why he didn't take his shoe off he says it was because it hurt too much to slide it over that big, red joint. Anyway, the adventure continues. Our friend spent dinner last night eating off other people's trays."

I stare at her.

She says, "He went around after he was done, into other people's room, checking out what they ordered and eating what was left. When one of the nurses stopped him and asked what he was doing, he said he was hungry. And when they told him they could order him more food, he said, "No, this is fine."

I get that feeling you sometimes have after hours of swimming, when you tip your head and suddenly there is more space in your ear (you mistakenly thought it was fine), and new sounds seem like new thoughts.

I say, "He's a little bizarre, isn't he?"

"Or really very hungry," Lynn answers.

"I'm going to tell him that he had another heart attack."

"Good luck," she says.

I walk down the hall, the light coming into patients' room bouncing off the silverware, the crosspieces of the IVs; everything arranged, even the temperature. All the faces a little sleepy. Finally quiet after a night of interruptions. Only movie-stars and the wives of politicians get rest when they go into hospitals.

As I walk down the hall I prepare myself. I try to think of how George will take his news. I try to count up his strengths and weaknesses, who he might have as supports in the world, his beliefs, but all I can think about is his wandering into other patients' rooms looking for scraps like some raccoon. I wonder if I should delay telling him the heart attack news until I straighten out this other problem, but six steps from his door, I decide not to wait: we need to move on with his care.

79

•

I had, earlier in my doctor life, presented bad news in what I thought was a kind and sad way. This way was comfortable for me. I decided what I would say before-hand almost to the word; I spoke softly. But not too softly because the patient would think their position was worse than it was and this would lower their morale. Of course, I wasn't overly optimistic either, because this was the mark of a charlatan and would only raise false hopes.

I've learned a few minor lessons over the years. I used to believe that small talk at times like these was in bad taste. But it isn't. If done before the news, it allows the patient to interrupt with the most frightening part of the big talk to come; small talk after the news allows patients to feel that things in life will go on. Small talk also allows me to give one of those grim but glimmering smiles which carry the truly important message: I have at least some feeling for what it must be like on the receiving end. I've also learned that some people prefer pessimism because it heightens the drama and gives them the chance of proving me wrong.

All this implies that I can imagine what it's like to be on the receiving end. I can't. It's the difference between one who recognizes the tune and one who knows the lyrics.

•

Although I call my work The White Life, in some ways I think of the hospital as dark. Darkness implies the unseen and that's how I imagine the sick live—puzzled, and in pervading obscurity. What is unseen? Roommates disappear, doctors conceal themselves in nonchalance. At home, we all become afraid at night, but in the hospital there is fear all day and night brings nothing new. Light brings its own terrors: new tests.

Over the years I have explained plenty of mysteries to patients: swellings, pains, discolorations, panic. I have heard them say, "I see." Just yesterday I told a man that he had lung cancer; "I see," he said. I understood for the very first time that this "seeing" was pure sensation; it had nothing to do with vision. It was sensation without meaning attached. The sick, the dying, already know they are sick or dying before I arrive.

My sons find on the ground during our walks what they know is there, what I miss. But when I give a name to what they find (just as I offer names for what my patients have found), something breaks and opens. My sons are always quiet after I speak.

Patients who receive bad news often go silent; they focus and dream at the same time. They sometimes don't answer to their name. And with a tremendous heave of spirit they become aware again. They see.

•

When I get to the door, George is sitting on the side of his bed, working on the breakfast tray that hangs off the end of his adjustable stand. I see the chipped white plate with its crimson border and the three-ball clump of eggs, cottage cheese and hash-browns (not your recommended cardiac diet, but who cares when more important things are afoot) and I try to think of clues I've missed about George that would tip me off about how best to reassure him. I wonder whether he will start to pace with news of his heart attack or simply withdraw and go numb. I remember his line about his pain being like spaghetti sauce, the first food analogy; I remember that he has no underwear with him, and his wanting to change rooms. None of these help me make guesses about George. Usually, with every day that passes, patients make themselves known to the doctor. It's like watching a Polaroid picture develop.

But Dittus is a negotiation between familiarity and strangeness. Despite sharing certain tics with my father, George is unlike him. George has a sense of difficulty about him. He has a sourness, and grimy fingers. He is more inward and alone and unavailable than I remember my father. In some ways, their resemblance bothers me. Memory is not always consolation.

"Juice, toast and a clear mind," Mr. Dittus says to me when I stand next to him. Then he says, "You figure out what's wrong with my foot?"

"Gout."

"Oh yeah, yeah," he says.

I had decided on the way in that George *did* have a clear mind, that I would give him the benefit of the doubt if he said anything strange to me. Therefore, anything he said that seemed fully rational would fit perfectly with my view of him and anything else could be discarded. It was much the way I viewed my son when he was a baby and sang his one note to the coffee grinder each morning, an event I took as a signal of talent; the babble and drool could be overlooked as I thought of his future.

I decide to take on George's wandering directly before proceeding to the bad news about his heart and then my medical plan.

"I heard that you were eating some extra dinners last night."

"Who told you that?" he asks angrily. "I was just visiting around and if people offer you something, you have to say yes."

"You can't go into other rooms," I tell him. "It annoys some people."

"Fine," he says.

My brilliantly conceived plans for delivering his bad news are now completely shot.

I sit down on the yellow chair next to him so we are at the same level. I say, "Let me catch you up on what's happened to you."

"That sounds bad," George says.

"Mostly I'm here to tell you that you've had another heart attack," I say. Do I say it softly, out of habit, out of a belief that if roommates hear bad news, they risk in some way being implicated? I'm not sure.

"That's a problem, I suppose," he says. He looks neither to his left nor to his right, but at my belt-line, indifferently. I am used to seeing puzzlement or anger or disappointment, some rearranging of the features. He doesn't even look sad.

"At the moment, it's not so much of a problem with you feeling so good," I say, trying to be optimistic. "Although your blood pressure is still high and may have to be controlled better."

"So I can go home?" he asks.

"We want to make sure you're safe to go home."

"Sure. Safe," he says sarcastically.

"You know, you were just here with the same problem two weeks ago."

"And they said, it wouldn't come back if I took care of myself. And I did take care of myself. All I did was some work around the house."

"I'm sure they mentioned you shouldn't do any heavy work for a little while after you left, didn't they?" I ask.

"I didn't."

"Weren't you scrubbing down your car when you got the pain?" I ask. I can feel myself blaming him, but it is mostly to get some rise out of him, some reaction I am familiar with. I feel badly doing it. Here I am, trained to give medical facts, to plan treatment, to discuss prognosis, to make decisions, and he's frustrating me. I want him to listen carefully, to be obedient, to survive. I see him as a willful man, a man who never loses his nerve, a sloppy man with unsuitable facial expressions, a man whose speech is nearly impossible to follow. A man who may be courageous or reckless, or courageous and reckless.

"So," he says.

"That counts as heavy work," I say.

"And I guess I should have been taking all the medicines they said. It probably would have helped if I got all those prescriptions filled too, right?"

"You weren't taking any medicines at home?" I ask. It is the first I've heard of this.

"I used what I had in the house."

"Did you tell anyone this since you've been here?"

"I don't think I did, come to think of it."

"What happened to your prescriptions?"

"I think they're on the counter in the bathroom. I was

feeling well. I was cured. I didn't think I needed them anymore."

It seems an even trade. I give him bad news, he gives me
bad news. Now I have to deal with why he hasn't been using
his medicines and what I am going to do about this in the
future. I shouldn't have expected anything different. There's
always a twist.

"Could you ask them to bring me some jello?" he asks,
and he picks up his spoon and looks down at his food again,
dismissing me.

•

George has a problem with his heart, the body's great
pump, its "main squeeze" my wife calls it, and yet I have
mentioned the flow of blood hardly at all. "The sight of
blood" is, purportedly, what keeps some people from
becoming doctors. On the other hand, extreme reactions to
blood, I suppose, may also attract some people to medicine,
just as sharks (the animal that brings blood to mind) attract
some people to scuba diving.

I remember the first time I found a patient's blood on me
thirty years ago. There is nothing as exhilarating and frightening as the blood of another person spurting on you. It was
the speed of it that I admired, the arc, the warm arrival. And
the fact that moments before it had passed by bone and muscle. As doctors, we pretend there is something natural about
blood, but outside the body there is nothing natural about it.
We, as doctors, may appreciate knowing that the inside can
be roused. We may even enjoy that it is so unlike water
(though we have been told what percentage of our make-up
is water—this includes blood—since grade school); it does
not reflect or ripple or wrinkle. But blood makes us nervous, if we let ourselves get nervous.

Age twenty-three, I was sitting across a patient's chest
like a bully when I felt that first blood on me. I was sitting
there pumping with the heels of my hands, trying to revive
him and his heart, this man with cirrhosis, my hands gloved
and his skin cool. I could feel his cartilage under my hands

and then he vomited blood and it began to soak into my pants and through to my skin. And when he was dead, I was told to use an opthalmoscope and look into the back of his eye, and still straddling him, I looked and saw where the blood had slowed so that it stacked; it bunched in black bands like burnt tortillas. More evidence that time had changed for this fellow. Moving blood reflects the time in our world, blood that does not move signals a different time.

When I left that room, still wet, and I saw his blood on me, I felt as if I were dragging this body across the floors of the hospital, bumping it along the ground, snagging it on corners; he was stuck to me, smearing the floor, leaving a trail, an inexhaustible supply of black from a hidden source.

When I took off my pants, the hairs on my legs were stuck together and red, the mark of Cain.

There is a line from Nietzsche: "There are occurrences of such a delicate nature that one does well to cover them up with some rudeness." That's how I've felt about blood since my first experience. Patients who bleed I still call, simply, rudely, "bleeders."

George has had heart attacks, in fact he's had great damage to that great blood pumper of his, and yet I have never seen George's blood.

•

On days when I don't get a new flood of patients, I teach my ward team in a conference room with a blackboard and chalk; this is called Attending Rounds; I am the Attending.

Why am I called an "Attending?" I don't know; perhaps in days past senior doctors *didn't* show up. "Rounds" is an historical term and refers to those days when doctors took their underlings around to see patients; most days we sit in the nurses' conference room with its crackers and brownies to discuss the business of the day, and we still call it Rounds.

Teaching gives me my greatest daily pleasure. I'll miss it when I leave. It's like my geologist friend discusses drilling for oil, bearing down through hard formation until you hit something soft and it begins to flow out, bubbling, their brains shining with discovery. Teaching pulls the interns and residents away from the bodies in the beds and lets them think in the abstract for an hour or two. Out on the wards, if my team does something wrong, it is my responsibility even if it's their fault or inattention. In the conference room, right and wrong don't matter so much.

Here's one way of thinking about how young doctors learn on the wards: Good judgment comes from experience; experience comes from bad judgment.

Sometimes I begin my hour-long conference by giving my team of residents and interns and medical students an abnormal test result, for instance a low blood count or a bad-looking X-ray. I ask my team what they'd do after receiving this report, and why. They always have to tell me why so I can watch them think. We go over the options and they want *all* of them. Youth. I say, "But you only get to choose one plan of attack, one confirmatory test or further diagnostic study." This limitation predictably makes them all moan. I want these students to go straight for what matters, then look around again. That is, think.

After they give me their choice for the next step, I ask, "And then what?" Or, "What if your first test choice doesn't give you any useful information?" I am relentless; I bother them. In general, my students and interns and residents become less pleasant-faced and mild-voiced, yet they remain, to a person, polite.

All this time I'm hoping that they see how uncertain this whole medical business is because (1) we're looking into the future and (2) it involves a patient, a person you don't really know, who makes decisions independent of us and whose body may or may not play by the rules.

Did I imagine that they would leave these Attending Rounds and go out and apply these lessons for more than three hours? Not in my most confident moments. But a few might.

Life is great until you weaken. I am weakening. I believe that my work is weakening me. There is evidence to this effect, truths I need to overlook in order to move through the day.

Medicine is all I know anymore, yet I have a fear of being only a doctor. This is a large fear. Strangely, to combat it I see more patients. I see more and more, hoping that in their rage and wisdom, they will teach me something.

This must sound crazy.

But take for example the next man I draw blood from. Neither of us will talk while I hurt him—the perpetrator and the victim always share a pact of silence. When it is over, he will give me some deep truth from his life, he will give me a secret. It always happens this way. But next time I fear it won't be enough.

What if he wants a secret from me? What if he wants me to tell him about myself? I won't be able to in any real way, and although I might make him relax or laugh our encounter will end on a sour note.

How could I, who despises needles, have come to be doing this? I do not tell this man that my major interest outside of medicine has always been skeets. The club I belong to is out in the country and has a clubhouse which is really just an empty cabin. It has a table, three cane chairs, a rusty little refrigerator and a bulletin board filled with NRA posters. My favorite says: Would HITLER have happened if the German public had the right to bear arms?

I go out into the field and load up two big red cartridges, each the size of a sausage, into my gun, and hold the butt tight to my shoulder and press the launcher with my toe. Twenty-five yards out, the little clay fucker tries to get away but turns to dust when it's hit. It makes me happy, the huge echo, the field sloping down, the quiet cloud of smoke hanging around for a while.

I am a sharpshooter and it doesn't take me long to reload a fresh one. Killing practice, I call it.

•

Why do I keep returning to George Dittus? He has none of the force and misery of the other patients I have this week. He doesn't want anything from me.

I pass George's room just before leaving the hospital. I hear a loud, two-fingered whistle as I go by. I look into his room and he motions me inside from his mustard yellow chair where he sits with his swollen toe up on the bed.

"Doc, nothing you could do for my foot," he says. "I knew it was gout. I've had gout. Nothing you could do."

"When did you last have it?" I ask.

"Come back some other time when you're not in a hurry somewhere," he says. He shoos me away.

Something has changed between us.

•

At home in bed, I get a call from an old friend, a woman I haven't spoken to in years who lives in a nearby state. Her mother lives in my town and has just been told that she has liver cancer. My old friend asks, "Who would you recommend as a doctor?" Since her mother has already been diagnosed, I figure that she already has a doctor and I ask who he or she is.

When I hear the name, I tell her, "He's pretty good." I immediately wish that I had said, "He's very good," and not been so ungenerous. He *was* very good from everything I knew about him. But really I'm no better than the average patient in judging a doctor whom I've never worked with. "I wouldn't switch," I tell her.

"That's a relief," she says. People hear what they want to hear.

"Do they know where the cancer originated?" I ask her.

"How would they know that?" she asks.

"They would have looked—a mammogram, checking your mother's colon."

"Would she know if they looked?"

I realize that this woman, a comparative literature pro-

88

fessor, my age, knows nothing about medicine. And why should she?

"What should I do to help her get things done?" she asks me.

"After a test, call to get the results. Then call again. Bug them. Doctors forget. Doctors don't call back. They don't confer frequently enough with each other either." I explain that doctors are often confusing because they are vaguely hostile. Bear with them.

I am speaking about myself.

I tell her, "You know Hippocrates said, 'Some patients recover through contentment with the goodness of their doctor.'"

When I hang up, I feel good. I feel like an insider. I understand that this is one of the major advantages of being a doctor, being able to help out friends.

I recently read an article in the *New York Times* about men and women becoming medical students after having another career. As I hunted down the continuation of this front page story in the crime-filled B-Section, I became envious of this second career group; the article returned me to my youth. I had gone directly from college to medical school to internship and residency with an impatient, ordering need, and I was clearly too young. But like others raised in the middle-class, concerned about slippage and without any particular physical, manual or intellectual skill, I chose medicine. Not out of great humanitarian impulse. Not out of lifelong obsessive interest or even much of an appreciation of the benefits. With no concern or understanding that my failure to strike out in original directions was evidence of a weak imagination. I knew, even at twenty-one years old, that doctors were societally guaranteed success.

Now, at the other end of a few years on the job, I have two thoughts about this guaranteed success. On the one hand, it represents long years of hard work and a good profession-picking sense and therefore I, and other doctors, deserve at least that respect. On the other hand, because doctors are individually replaceable, and take a risk-free career path compared to one such as professional sports where only a few people make it big—here I must take a deep breath before making a loony assertion—doctors are absurdly overpaid.

I was envious of those in the *New York Times* article until I realized that they had probably failed at or lost interest in some career, and this must have had a rebuking effect on them. As a doctor, you never fail unless you commit suicide or do drugs *and* get caught. I was envious until I realized that not only were these people in their thirties starting out again, taking on debt, unloading previously-supported kids on spouses, but in general they also did not know what they were in for (the waiting and looking and believing and getting fooled), even with another career behind them. Then the article's reporter put in this bit about a TV producer who was starting medical school because she had been out on a shoot with a physician who happens to notice a drowning child, dives into what was to be the backdrop lake, drags the kid out and saves her with CPR. What this had to do with becoming a doctor confused me. All you needed were swimming lessons and a CPR course, which my wife had just taken at the local Red Cross chapter, in order to save our children and me if the need arose. But somehow this all got translated into the need for the producer to go to medical school.

•

What happens when a doctor writes in the ORDERS section of a patient's chart, 'Please send for stress test,' as I do in George's chart on Wednesday morning? Orders, in this case, means commands. The unit secretary finds a chart with new Orders in it on his/her desk, calls that part of the hospital which schedules the commanded test, and tells the nurse (and sometimes the doctor) when the patient should get their shoes on and go.

In a stress test, the patient is rolled in a wheelchair by one of the hospital's "transporters" to the hospital's second floor. Transporters are badly paid, but instructed by their supervisors to be kind to patients, smile, and drive slowly. Transporters wear white pants and surgical scrub shirts. Most, men and women, also wear at least one earring. Transporters speak only to each other, take long lunch breaks, and walk *unbelievably* slowly. Many have been on the transport team for years and seem to enjoy their work. It's too bad that transporters can't live up to their names. It's too bad they can't put you in their chair and take you someplace sublime.

On the second floor, in the stress test suite (rooms are called suites, just as pet cages are sometimes called crates by veterenarians as a means of subterfuge), a technician places electrodes on the chest of the patient to monitor the heart rhythm, and then asks him to walk on a treadmill.

Doctors generally think of test results in binary terms: abnormal/normal, positive/negative. Such results seem understandable and unmistakeable, but when I tell my team that such terms disguise more complex meanings, that life is never as simple as that, there is audible head-scratching and much eye-rolling. Doctors think in binary terms, but they do not *speak* this way with patients. Anyone who has ever been to see a doctor knows that the medically-trained always use "maybes," or "if things go fine," or "there are a number of possibilities"; the obligatory qualifiers get inserted even after a rave review of your physical condition. If things are bad, there is cautious hope that leaves room for heroism. Doctors hedge. It's paradoxical then that this shading is the opposite of how test results get interpreted. But I'd submit that in many cases test results are not always so clear.

The risks of the binary approach are (1) when a doctor calls a test (such as a stress test) "positive" (which leads to patient anxiety, changes on insurance policies, and a chain of explanations) it may be *falsely* positive (as a result of technical error or the interference of assorted factors sometimes called imperfection), and thus the doctor may be wrong and, (2) when a doctor calls a test "negative" (leading to relief and, often, feelings of invulnerability with the resumption of bad habits) it may be *falsely* negative (for the same reasons as before) and again the doctor may be wrong. These "falsies" are not infrequent and do not suggest that the doctor is doing a second-rate job of testing or interpreting. They simply imply that *all* medical tests are imperfect. When I first explained these risks to my ward team of young doctors, there was great disappointment. Deep down, perhaps they didn't believe me; there is comfort in the binary approach to life.

Sharing uncertainty (which is absent from the binary approach) with patients has good and bad sides, no doubt. Telling patients about uncertainties (in the simplest case, the risk of a medication's side effects) may scare them enough to refuse the pill that you, as doctor, believe is in their best interest. Therefore, some doctors feel that it is just a waste of time to have these discussions. On the other hand, if uncertainties are not explained, expectations may be set that are unrealistic, and potentially haunting for all involved. I recommend to my students sharing their uncertainty. At least most of the time, and certainly if a patient wants honesty.

•

I decide to return to my office to read my mail. I realize that I've given no hints about what my office looks like other than that there is a photograph of a tattooed man on the wall. With the door shut, my office is about ten-by-fourteen feet, with my maroon desk along the wall between the door and the waist high window. As I sit at my desk, to my right out the window is half a parking lot.

If you look around in my office you would never know that I am a doctor. There is a bookcase that has some unmarked binders filled with the materials of courses I've taught. There is a standing file, closed and unlabeled, that holds old manuscripts, and medical journal articles arranged by subject: Heart Failure, Hepatitis, et cetera. In the corner, next to my desk, there is a small round cherry table covered with unanswered correspondence. One white coat hangs from the peg by my door, but this might just as well belong to a freezer repairman. If I sit at my desk and look over my computer, I can stare at my photograph of the tattooed man. I have no diplomas on the walls in black frames, I have no oversized textbooks, I have no visible reflex hammer.

The decision to work with your door open or closed is the essential question of all office politics. Open allows you to snoop, and to overhear conversations, and get the first look at visitors (at which point you can get up—if you are fast—and close the door). Open allows the eye-up interruption of people passing; the voyeur brain associates a flash of dress or trouser-shoe border with an office-mate and this pause permits a reconstitution of thought on the work at hand as well as an idea of who to have lunch with that day. Clearly, less work gets done with an open door policy. Closing your door signals snobbery, unfriendliness, secrets.

I usually close my door when I come in in the morning and when I leave my office a half hour later to see patients on my five-by-eight cards, I prop my door open: welcome, I'm not in, you're welcome to enter.

When I leave my office, checking Marie's latest work over her shoulder, I always pass the coffee room with self-doubt. I have not given to the coffee fund because I drink coffee only once or twice a year (our coffee tastes like every muffler-shop waiting room brand with its carbon-dated Coffee-Mate), but I know this stinginess is ignoble and bad for my reputation. I have never been asked about my contribution (or lack of a contribution) after the initial memo requesting seventy-five dollars for the year, but I am sure every doctor and administrator and secretary who uses this room remembers my "oversight"; if I see any coffee drinkers in that room I feel badly and I could not speak with them there; outside that room, if they carry their soft cups to their offices, they are just my colleagues.

•

Although I make a big deal, when teaching my students, about considering many diagnoses and choosing the appropriate test to narrow your list, and I downplay the need for the immediate gratification of a "right answer," the truth is I love to make The Diagnosis. Although I've made two thousand of them before, I still find myself excited in the first moments after I figure it out. It's like reeling in a fish. You do it inch by inch believing nearly the whole time that it's a weed or a stick under there, but still reeling because you remember that first little twitch, that jump on the line, and it makes you an optimist. When it breaks water and you see the flapping truth you've reached the ultimate moment. When you can say the name and get ready to tell others, when you know it won't be a secret for long.

The best diagnosis is when you have no more information than what you see or hear from the patient, or in the patient. When you can say (before ordering any test), "I know what's going on in there."

•

All that matters to the patient is what you find wrong with them. I am not sure what to say to Mr. Dittus, what the right approach is in order to convince him to have a stress test. Should I use the measured, unsurprising binary (but discretely qualified) method, or the turmoil-ridden approach that can be forgiven because it invites questions and shares responsibility? On the way down the hall I give myself a review. Try to avoid the pretend-scholarly; don't rubber-band your ideas, give them one at a time; talk slowly. And most of all: stop and ask for questions in order to avoid the mutual deafness that characterizes most doctor-patient talk.

I walk into Mr. Dittus's room. It smells of air freshener and heat.

"How are you feeling?" I ask him. He is twisting and turning as usual and I cannot get a good look at his eyes. His eyes don't stay put. They do not behave.

"How are you feeling?" he answers. Patients never ask how I am. They have their own problems. But he is unashamedly direct.

"Not enough time in the day to read the paper," I tell him. When I'm on the wards, I go weeks without anything more than a glance at the front page.

"I don't have enough interest in the present to read a newspaper," he says. "My mother read the paper every day. Roley on her lap. Roley was her dog, old wheezy mutt-terrier. He slept on her lap. He ate off of her plate."

I sit down in the yellow chair. I see that I'm going to be a while. At first, George wouldn't talk. Now he doesn't let me leave.

"He had a head like a lopsided apple. Like one of those apples you pick off the ground but that you just throw down somewhere. I know why you're tired all the time," he informs me. "Same as I was, no sleep. All my jobs were night jobs, hours that would kill most people. When I took tickets on the turnpike, I used to sit in that box that was no bigger than a telephone booth. I wore slippers. If you're up all night, might as well wear slippers, I say. About eleven o'clock some nights I got restless, but I couldn't leave that little room. And too many nasty people driving by so I quit and went into security. But you meet nice people at night, printers, firemen. Never meet doctors though. You're here. If you work at night you never want to see anyone during the day though."

"I think you should probably have a stress test, a test to see if you're at risk for more heart attacks," I tell him. Just like that.

"Are you the boss?'

"Yes," I say.

"Just making sure," Mr. Dittus said. "You know, some days it's chickens and some days it's feathers."

I have no idea what this means.

I start again. "So a stress test is a test where you walk and we monitor your heart and . . . "

"No. I don't think so," George says.

His tone is not far from scolding.

"No stresses. Not now," George tells me in his friendliest voice. He rubs his hands together. I'm trying to solve a problem that isn't a problem, I figure he is thinking. He is more confident about his future than I am, and this stymies me.

Mr. Dittus is silent. Then he says, "You know, my foot still hurts."

"I'm worried about your heart," I tell him.

"What can I do? I'm obliged to live with myself," he tells me. He looks down at his red palms.

How hard do I push? Not hard.

George is ignorant of his risk. But his ignorance has the force of feeling. I believe that he also distrusts what can be physically known.

•

Can I explain to my students in one sentence what this doctoring job is about? They need simple direction. I try to tell them about Realists and People of the Imagination, which is meant as a parable about us and George, about doctors and the patients to whom they've given bad news. I tell them, Realists advise: Open your eyes and look. People of the Imagination advise: Close your eyes to see better. The doctor's job is to have these two truths meet, to come up with a plan.

My students have no idea what I am talking about.

•

I go down the hall in search of other patients to see. I pass rooms of quadriplegics, motionless, restful, absorbent, living in memories of motorcycle trauma, springboard accidents. I think of their bodies and the usual rules of nature: soft within, rigid without. Except us. Humans. Vulnerable, injured by cold and heat and force. No shell, hide, scales, bristles. That the old are frayed, leveled by injury, bloodied, is no surprise. But the quadriplegics bother me.

The chorus in Greek tragedies often found themselves powerless before events. So they sought not solutions, but expressions of what happened. This is how I feel passing the quadriplegics.

I think of my own dreams of the future and how useful they are. For the quads, in my mind at least, the present presses, just getting through it. After years in beds and chairs, I wonder what they dream about.

Time dominates in the hospital. Or rather, a variety of times do. Most often time is mechanical as we doctors sit at nurses' stations, writing in charts, waiting for patients' tests to finish. In the morning, the halls are miraculously cleared like a city emptied of people, the hospital seems like a drowsy place. But then, emergencies happen. Time becomes dense and abrupt, a woman found pulseless. A sudden rush. Adrenaline. The unforseeable and fleeting.

Maybe this variation in pace is why the clocks on the walls of the hospital are never in agreement. Patients tell their stories to stop time, for the story of illness includes life Before Telling.

Police also work on stop and go time. Walk into any station in any town or city, and you'll see men (occasionally women) sitting around, reclining. But you also know that things get done when they have to. When I've been in big city stations, I know that I am with people who see more tragedy in a day than most people do in a lifetime. I know that I am with people who, after a few years, consider the dead body less important than what's happening after work. I know that I am with people who not only want successes, but want instant successes, who usually have no patience. I know that I am with people who think they are going out of their way to give you a full explanation, while I'm thinking: Out of what way?

•

The familiar signs on the walls keep me moving: HOUSEKEEPING, PHARMACY SATELLITE, LINEN ROOM, PATIENT AREA—QUIET PLEASE, OPEN

DOOR SLOWLY. Leaving 9A, I pass the old man harnessed to his chair, the same man in every hospital, his hands tilting and gliding, yelling at something invisible, "Watch him. He's coming in for a landing."

I find one of my patients on the far end of 9B, a fifty-two-year-old woman who has been awakened by tingling in her hand and foot. She was admitted in order to check whether she had had a stroke. But now, forty-eight hours after her admission, she still has these same complaints and we have no answers for her. After I review my meager findings with her and admit my ignorance, I ask her, "Is anything unusual going on at home?"

Her face colors. Anger comes up in her eyes. She says, "You wouldn't ask that if I were a man." She has a lipless mouth and sweet breath.

I say, "Yes I would." And indeed I had when questioning Mr. Dittus.

"Sorry if I'm skeptical, but you wouldn't," she tells me. We are quiet for a moment. I am baffled; she is fierce.

"You know, when I came in here I considered not telling people, I didn't tell anyone, that I was on an antidepressant, that I'd been treated for depression because they, you, would see me in a certain way."

"How's that?" I ask.

"Like I wasn't really . . . Never mind."

She starts crying.

"I'm glad I live with my son," she says, "because when I woke up it started spreading up my hands to my arms, my feet to my legs, and I couldn't get back from the bathroom. I just couldn't move. I was scared. I couldn't move even to the telephone, so I called him. I knew he would take care of me. And when I got here I wasn't going to tell anyone because of getting questions like you just asked."

"I didn't know that you took antidepressants," I say.

"They why did you ask about my home?"

"I asked you what I ask everyone whose symptoms I can't put into a little box."

"Even men?"

"Even men. I just did in fact."

"And what answer did you expect from me?"

"Expect?"

"Would you be looking for to give you something valuable."

"Most any answer is helpful," I tell her, and this is true. Her crying itself is helpful. We go back and forth like this a while longer until our conversation dwindles away into quiet again. I still have no answer for her, and I feel bad for her. I am not a tribunal, I want to say. But I don't believe that I can explain this to her. In the end, I offer her only the reassurance that we have found nothing awful to explain her symptoms.

Although my question was not sexist, it was taken in that spirit. Had I presented it poorly or was I kidding myself? Was there a way I could have spoken to her without angering her? I believe that this has nothing to do with sexism, but rather with my whole approach to patients and uncertainty. I demand revelation. Perhaps I am too harsh.

I need to quit. I need a vacation, a new job.

In the hall I remember a passage in Herodotus: "They bring out the sick to the marketplace. People who walk by, and have suffered the same ill as the sick man's, or seen others in like cases, come near and advise him about his disease and comfort him, telling him by what means they have themselves recovered of it, or seen others to recover. None may pass by the sick man without speaking and asking what is his sickness."

My patient needs someone who will tell her how they recovered.

People moving through the world are often heartbroken but not aware of it; here, they are always aware of it.

•

I know the hall of 9A well. It is usually a peaceful floor with good nurses. I know which of them are exuberant and which are pessimistic. I know the sounds: the katydids of the monitors. It's my city: explorable and haphazard, enclosed and finite and therefore lonely.

George whistles me down again when I pass his room.

"Sorry to say no to your stress test, Doc," he says. "Here's my foot." He wriggles his bare toes at me. "Thought you'd want to see it again soon."

I should try hard with George now, I've decided. He's ambushed me and as a famous journalist once said, "The one thing about being ambushed is that you can never take yourself very seriously again." I try hard to be serious and concentrated. But I smile when I see George's chaotic face, his chewed ears, his tongue rubbing the inside of his cheek. His shirt is open, his red hair is a mess, he looks as if he'd been to an all-night party.

"Thanks," I say. "But this is only a social call." Some visits with doctors may seem to be social, but they're not, exactly.

"You remind me of my mother," George tells me.

"Thanks," I say. "How's that?"

"The way you apologized. She always apologized when I caught her up to something. That's the last time I had gout. When my mother was alive."

"She live around here?"

"You remember I told you about working as a security guard?"

I can only imagine him as unemployed, a man who dodges bill collectors.

"Some people say you have to be patient to be a security guard, but truth is you just have to be lazy," George tells me.

"Ever have a break-in?" I ask.

"The place where I worked had fences that were fifteen feet high. You kidding? They didn't need me. But I walked around a lot. On my feet all night. And one morning I got home and my mother noticed that my foot swelled up."

"She was living with you?"

"I was living with her."

"Around here?"

"I didn't want to live with her, but who else would? I was all the family she had. 'I need some human company,' she was always telling me, so I moved in."

"Your father?"

"My father wore suspenders and was baptized twice, that should tell you who *he* was. He made dentures for a living. It killed him. Anyway, she was always talking about her Bible, what she was reading in her Bible. I couldn't give two nits about her Bible. Heaven and Hell; I didn't want to go to either—they both sounded awful. She saw my red toe and wanted to pour liquor on it. She used to drink you know."

"I didn't know," I tell him.

"Drank her beer and sang hymns at the same time. If it had ice in it, it wasn't liquor according to her. She liked to sing. 'A little tweet,' my father called her. Ever been in a car crash?"

"No," I answer.

"I have. That's what gout feels like. I don't know how she saw my foot with the room so dark. She kept her rooms dark. She had these yellow curtains over the lamps. I guess she had good eyes."

My beeper goes off. "Excuse me," I say.

"Do your business," he says. "And keep your eyes open."

•

It's a call to see another patient and as I take the stairs to the seventh floor, I suddenly remember Mr. Dittus telling me that he never took the medicines that had been prescribed after his first heart attack. I had ignored this tidbit and thereby suppressed the obvious conclusion that his disinterest in pills was central to his care at this point. Taking these medications might well have prevented this second heart attack. For the second time I consider involving our social work department to help us sort out George's various reluctances.

I stop at the phone by the 7B clerk's desk. On the counter is a pile of mail, clutched by a rubber band, ready to be delivered. Hospitals are probably the only places other than jails where people still write letters. (On vacations, people now send postcards; I'm surprised hotels even leave a few sheets of stationary in the bedside drawer anymore.) It's strange to think that jails, hospitals and vacation spots are probably the only places where the sights are varied enough and the feelings worthy enough to warrant correspondence.

I call the Social Work department, leaving a message with my name, Mr. Dittus's name and the reason that I need help.

•

Lunch in the hospital cafeteria is my favorite time of the day. Moving my still-wet-from-the-awfully-big-dishwasher green tray (I always choose green over red or blue) along the horizontal silver parallel bars is completely satisfying. If you believe that you can learn everything about a person by finding out his or her notion of what a truly happy life would be, pushing a green tray and selecting my lunch from behind steamy glass is my answer.

I love the macaroni and cheese. Thick, sun-yellow, glutinous. It is offered in a serve-yourself stainless steel casserole dish near the salad bar. I pay by weight. Sometimes I also take a little salad for my health. Chocolate pudding for dessert.

The seating in our cafeteria is a slightly less awkward version of what you'd find in any high school cafeteria: nurses sit with nurses, risk managers sit with risk managers, respiratory therapists eat together, secretaries join other secretaries. The room is the size of a small airplane hangar (our hospital is the largest employer in the state), with seventy-foot ceilings and a small, enclosed herbarium in the middle of things. The tables are long and brown with hundreds of identical salt and pepper shakers, and little standing cardboard triangles, spaced every two tables, promoting new hospital activities: the weight-loss program, an employee bus-trip to Atlantic City, a reminder that it is secretary's week. The doctors retreat to the back and sit at four round tables. I generally sit with the surgeons.

My decision during medical school not to become a surgeon was simple. I was afraid of those extra holes cut in the body, the skin parting and opening under the false lights just seemed wrong to me, terrifying. The patient's face, expressionless beyond the curtain and our hands inside their body. Blood from some faraway red melt pouring out, swirling; the tissues shining, fat coming unstuck. Organs, pockets, swollen patterns, flaps, slits, tiny suctions, laws I didn't know, laws that had been concealed were now revealed in this De Kooning clutter. During each surgery I thought: I don't know what's going on here; I have no idea.

The surgeons I met during medical school never thought this, not for a minute. To them, surgery was a long, brute game. I suppose being a surgeon is like being a stunt pilot— if you notice how you feel, you can't do the work.

The surgeons whom I eat lunch with are an older group. They are boys gone gray, clear-eyed, attentive. They have known each other for years. They have common references. Dressed in their blue scrubs with paper shoe-coverings, they talk about their interesting operations from that week. They talk, for instance, about the kid flown in from The Island after getting thrown from a scooter. Massive internal blood loss. This leads to talk of The Island itself, thirty miles off-shore and a summer escape, which leads to the subject of boats and where one could refuel on The Island, to where they keep their boats during the winter, to the power of various motors, to who they use to clean the hulls. To the cost of a boat's upkeep. Not having a boat, not even knowing how to sail, leaves me as an outsider who smiles and nods his head a lot. As when they speak of their work, these surgeons are loud and gruff offering their dazzling, free-of-fact opinions. Still, it seems that all the extraordinary events of the world are missing from our lunch-time conversations:

wars, elections, state politics. The cost of motors leads inevitably to the most recent damage to their incomes.

They let me sit in, they let me listen even to this private talk of dollars perhaps because I never join in the complaining. There is no good news to be found for them. Once cafeteria despots, they have become great, disappointed individualists whining. Never for a moment do they think: we make so much more money than this internist among us. They deserved what they got. Eating hamburgers and salads and ice creams, their eyes roll with each new problem discussed. The good old days, the unknowably hard work, their overgenerous (family-depriving) attention to patients, were gone. They practiced according to strict, abstract standards, clear material directives about success, and it had come to this. I remember about those surgeons from the 1500's, how they got paid only if the patient was cured, how they lived in the patient's house awaiting the outcome. Here I am, four hundred years later, with the knights of the last generation at their round table and their benevolent attitude has disappeared; they have been lowered, left dissatisfied, left to clutch and rattle the past.

I appreciate their hustle and theatrical talk and enormous pride. I'm beginning to think like they do. This is dangerous ground.

Surgeons are people who know how to refold maps, whereas I get lost without noticing.

•

Carrying my tray to the conveyor which carries my paper-free leftovers into the hidden kitchen, I get paged by Peg from Social Work.

I walk over to my office before I call her back.

"I'm supposed to see a friend of yours, a Mr. George Dittus," Peg says. "What's the scoop?"

"The scoop is two heart attacks in two weeks, not much insight into his heart disease and noncompliance. He also doesn't want a stress test or anything to do with my suggestions."

"Non-compliance," Peg says, real slowly. I could hear an in-breath of disgust. I had used one of those words which had lost its meaning from overuse and I am ashamed. "And by that you mean . . . ?"

"After he left the last time, he never took his pills. He thought he was cured. Never even filled the prescription."

"What's he do all day?" Peg asks.

Social workers focus on questions like these that doctors usually have little time for, or, more accurately, interest in. If we learn a patient's job-title, we rarely ask what this work actually involves; only if a patient does something truly bizarre (loading mercury into thermometers, cleaning sewers) do we believe that it might, *might*, have something to do with Disease. "I don't know," I tell her. I know a lot about George, but not this.

"Did he used to work?" she asks.

"As a security guard. But I don't know when he gave it up or what he's done since." I imagine him as a bellhop, a small-time fight promoter, a war refugee, a school dropout, a teenage runaway, but I have never asked him directly about his current job. All I know is that he gets by on a slim Social Security payment.

"Does he live with anyone?"

"I think he lived with his mother, but she died, I don't know when. I don't think he lives with anybody now," I tell her. Again, I'm not sure though.

"Any family?"

"He says none."

She keeps asking me questions I can not answer, important questions I understand it is worth knowing the answers to. Peg is tough on anything that smacks of vagueness. She is irresistible on a certain level. Pudgy and clever.

"He must have just come in," she says, offering me an excuse for my ignorance.

"Day three," I tell her. I hear another long breath. Peg is tired of doctors. I know she considers us Ad-men, simplifying patients into that single, instantly recognizable advertisment: a diagnosis. She is even disappointed in me, and the longer I speak with her the more I become disappointed in myself.

Social workers are a paradox to me: they have a sense of themselves as being non-judgmental and accepting, yet they pass judgment quicker than anyone. They make my wife look slow. There is another contrast in Peg. She has a huge voice, a magnificent, intimidating voice and yet she stands at only four foot nine—although her curly hair gives her a few more inches.

"Does he have medical insurance? Maybe that's why he didn't fill his prescriptions," Peg reasonably asks.

"I don't know what insurance he has," I tell her.

And then I tell Peg something about George that is also true about me these days.

"He's a little agitated in a way he can't contain," I say.

"I see," she says. "And when are you planning to send him home?" Which means: do I have to see him today?

"I hope in a few days," I say. "After I convince him that two heart attacks is enough." I also say, "Thanks," which actually impresses Peg.

•

When I hang up, I see a new patient. She is a fifty-five-year-old woman, legally blind from diabetes. She has adopted her granddaughter who is six-years-old, whose mother is a heroin addict. The girl's father sometimes lives in the house as well; I'm told he's unpredictable and prone to violence, although never directed at the family. My fifty-five-year-old-patient has her granddaughter draw up the insulin into a syringe twice a day for her because she can't see. She has visiting nurses come in weekly to check on things but they complain that at those visits all the necessary insulin injection supplies (needles, syringes, alcohol wipes, the insulin itself) are never there. My patient comes in with her blood sugar out of control, feeling washed out, no surprise. She drove to the hospital, her grandaughter, who could see, steering. Six hours later she is feeling better and wants to leave. She wants to eat dinner at home. This is how people live. I'm still not sure how I missed George's foot; it still bothers me. I had somehow lost track of my ritual examination, down the body from the top, a ritual that protected me (and patients) and made me feel competent and proud, perhaps even kept me happy. I had lost that ritual during my time with George.

•

The index card on the top of my pile is Mr. Elderkin's. At eighty-nine, the exact day, the exact month has slipped away from him. Most times, he knows that he's in a hospital, although sometimes he thinks our hospital is in North Carolina. He has no idea what is wrong with him and he doesn't remember that his son dropped him off a week before and disappeared. His son does not have a phone, and doesn't have an address that he tells anyone, but he does have a deaf and mute girlfriend (also in her fifties) who wears print miniskirts and black leggings and who the son sends in to visit (although she never divulges his address). I have the sense in talking with Mr. Elderkin that he knows something bad is happening although he isn't sure it is happening to him. Actually, he has lung cancer. He is weak, unable to walk and can't go back to living alone. Where can he go? To the son who never visits him? He refuses to consider any possibility other than living alone, and nursing homes won't consider him unless he will consider them; he won't. Using the words "nursing home" with Mr. Elderkin puts him in a bad mood. Nursing homes know about this image problem and have begun calling themselves by other names: convalescent villages or retirement parks. Patients always understand that we are talking about nursing homes. Habit being so strong, Mr. Elderkin thanks me for raising the subject even as it puts him in a bad mood. He just sits in his room, and the social worker, a colleague of Peg's who got involved early on, keeps calling the police to ask them to go out and find Mr. Elderkin's son so we can ask him some questions about his father's future care.

Then I go to see a Cambodian man who has mistakenly overdosed on aspirin by taking too much Nyquil, a pregnant woman whose asthma was triggered when she vacuumed her dusty carpet, and a ninety-three-year-old, slightly demented man with a German accent and a pneumonia who had been the object of a triage battle down in the Emergency Room. I had heard that in the Emergency Room he claimed to be a war veteran, and so the staff (after seeing that his condition was stable) put him in an ambulance and set him across town to the Veteran's Hospital. They attached a card to his hospital gown that read: World War I vet. He had come back to our hospital about six hours later with another card on his chest: Right War, Wrong side. Mr. Ochman had been in the *German* army and the Vet's Hospital saw no reason to treat him as one of their own.

After an hour of these visits, I have grown tired of amazing things.

I drive across town to the university pool, which is open Wednesday evenings, and go swimming. Thankfully, the lanes run across and not the lengthwise fifty meters which give me that sinking feeling. I swim fast and look at the college girls underwater as they let me pass. There is no hot water in the shower after I do my usual twenty minutes. There is a man with only a single leg who balances easily on his one thong.

•

I like when they call me doctor. I like the sound of it.

I resent that non-medical people have begun calling themselves doctor. I blame this phenomenon on the book *Dr. Doolittle*.

This is how Dr. Doolittle begins: "Once upon a time, many years ago—when our grandfathers were little children—there was a doctor; and his name was Doolittle—John Doolittle, M.D.. "M.D." means that he was a proper doctor and knew a whole lot."

The spreading of "doctor" can be linked to John Doolittle, who loved pets and who "got more and more animals; the people who came to see him got less and less." From the same book: "As a matter of fact, it takes a much cleverer man to be a really good animal-doctor than it does to be a good people doctor." This was the beginning of the end for the term "doctor," which no longer had anything to do with taking care of people.

Now everyone calls themselves doctor. There are tree doctors, car doctors, spin doctors, there is Dr. J. Even dentists call themselves doctors. I reject this and consider it unmannerly. Not very many things work me up like this. When I look in our Yellow Pages, there is no one listed under Doctor. We're under "Physicians," a word I despise and believe was invented only because of everyone calling themselves doctors.

It feels good to defend doctors once in a while. As one of my lunch-time surgeons said to me today while discussing last week's medicine-pounding segment of *Sixty Minutes: A Weekly News Magazine:* "If they left doctors alone, they could call it *Thirty Minutes*."

•

In bed, watching television, I realize: What George is to me is no more than my father was to Dr. Gresser. A patient for whom I feel a helpless but limited empathy. A difficult man with his own opinions.

•

In addition to those patients that I have to see on ward duty, there are those patients I would like to have, whom I imagine having under my care. I remember spying Norman Mailer in a supermarket one summer. I watched him push his cart, bow-legged in khaki shorts, smaller than I figured, and getting old. He had an ace-wrap around his left knee, a slight limp. I saw what he had in his basket—B &M Baked Beans, oranges, paper towels—but I kept thinking: who is his doctor? What's wrong with his knee? Part of me wanted to speak with him, take his history (now that would be a great history to take), but I didn't want to intrude. I was sure that he was always accosted; let the poor old guy shop, I thought.

His knee was clearly bothering him. I followed him, at a distance, to check-out. I watched him over the bank of candy. In order to pay, he started to tell the checker his charge number. But half way through, he forgot the last digits. He stood in front of me cursing himself, wondering aloud what had happened to those last numbers, until the checker sent him off, another old man with cheeks red as a spanking and a failing mind, over to the information desk to let someone help him look it up. Did this mean that Mailer's memory was shot? Had he had it checked out? And what was the story he would tell his doctor about this supermarket visit? Would he even mention it? I couldn't remember a doctor in one of his books. What did he think of them? He was probably unimpressed; therefore the omission. But more importantly, what would he think of me?

Some authors I would want to avoid having as patients. I never want William Styron visiting my office. This is what he wrote on page 44 of *Darkness Visible*, his diary of depression. "I made the reckless mistake of downing a scotch and soda—my first alcohol in months—which sent me into a tailspin, causing me such a horrified sense of disease and interior doom that the very next day I rushed to a Manhattan internist, who initiated a long series of tests . . . After three weeks of high-tech and extremely expensive evaluation, the doctor pronounced me totally fit."

Does Styron really expect a sophisticated reader, especially one who practices medicine, to believe this absurd and incomplete account? The most reckless mistake in his retelling (in all likelihood a novelist's lie) is of course the last line, because there is no doctor who will pronounce a patient "totally fit." It may be that this summation is Styron's twisting, interpretive style; he meant simply that *he* felt better at the end of the visit.

But the entire description of this episode is unbelievable. Notice what we don't get from this account and you begin to understand why I appreciate patients like George Dittus and why I wish never to see Bill Styron. First: we don't know what Styron complained of during his doctor visit, which means we don't know if the tests ordered were appropriate. "High-tech" is a code word; it suggests that the tests were unnecessary. Second: we don't know if Styron told his doctor that he drank alcohol the day before, or even if the doctor asked. Third: had Styron ever seen this doctor before? And if so, did this doctor know about his history of depression, which is obviously relevant to number two above.

All we know for sure, it seems to me, is that Styron was seen the day after his "tailspin" began. This seems like pretty good service for a non-emergency in Manhattan. (If it were an emergency I assume he would have gone to an emergency room.)

Am I overreacting here? After all, the book is about one man's depression, not about the medical profession. Why get hung up on this one paragraph? Why do I resent this writing so much given all my own pouncing on fellow doctors? Partly because Styron, who approaches all his books in search of some moral pill, here won't let his doctors prescribe much at all. But mainly, I'm upset by this typically sloppy thinking about doctors by likable-seeming, intelligent people. In fact, I'd go as far as to say: you can't trust most people writing about their own illness. They lie or give only a few of the facts. Which is not to say that illness books can't be inspiring; like television docudramas, you believe what you're seeing even though all the details are wrong.

•

When I wake up on Thursday morning, I can't move my neck. I try turning to my right to kiss my wife when a pain drives south along my spine turning left into my shoulder-blade. As an experiment, I try turning to the left to look out the window. I can't move that way either without ice-pick pain in the other scapula. I lay staring at the ceiling, silent, enjoying the keen pleasure of painlessness for a moment until I become angry and self-blaming. I can't think of what I've done to myself to bring on this problem and I've never had an immobilizing pain like this in my neck before. I say nothing to my wife whom I feel against my right leg pivoting easily toward me, readying for our ritual AM smooch in the moments before the little volcanoes with legs next door wake up and come rushing in and onto us.

My first ceiling thoughts are a review of the diagnostic possibilities which I pursue with a bodily hypervigilance and a professional rigor. I have heard those cartilaginous clicks in my neck for months while playing tennis and I have even begun taking a prophylactic aspirin before hitting the courts recently. But this neck-noise-nuisance I attributed to simple aging, and there have been no recent changes in my game; my partners are the same, I still sweat and lose valiantly. I have not slept badly nor did I find myself at midnight in some awkward dream-induced contortion. Sex is a dead-solid absolute bet not to be the cause of this pain. Although I consider cancer metastatic to my vertebrae (which would mean imminent death, dying being the immediate concern of anyone who feels in any way ill and which is at the root of every doctor-patient conversation, even visits for colds), I feel sure that my neck muscles are simply and powerfully in spasm. Nothing more serious than that. But when I hear my wife say, "Kiss me," and I try again to move without success, all I can do is pull the covers over my head like a hunchback in an overcoat. From under there, I explain the problem to her, that my behavior has nothing to do with not wanting to kiss her, whereupon she goes (so easily, so freely) to get me some aspirin and to tell the boys to keep off my neck.

My family often tells me that I do not believe in American medicine, its faith in progress and remedies. They tell me that I say to them, as often as not, "That problem of yours will go away on its own. Leave it alone." As a general approach, this is true about me, though I'm not sure if it can be taken as a sign of optimism or of pessimism, or as evidence that I like to think mostly about good things, not failure, or rather that as a doctor I quickly developed an ignore-it attitude toward potential catastrophe. Of course, I am not wholly nihilistic, which would represent as deep an irony as the decal on a sixteen-wheeler that recently filled my rear-view mirror for a mile before passing me, PLEASE DRIVE SAFELY. So I take the aspirin she brings me.

I do not have a doctor of my own. I waver about whether this is appropriate. Most times I believe that I do not need a regular doctor given my lack of chronic health problems, and the low probability of developing one at my still-youthful age. In this, I am like most American males, who not only believe they don't need a doctor, but don't have one. On the other hand, I am a primary care doctor, the type of doctor whose very mission it is to convince others (including my students) that everyone should have a doctor who can give them routine care, or who can be contacted should a problem arise.

The doctors I know take care of themselves, serve as their own doctors, just like other people. Doctors aren't much interested in teaching other people to take care of themselves though. Patients know this and have taken matters into their own hands. They barely need us anymore. I recently counted 240 do-it-yourself test kits in my neighborhood pharmacy. If you can do it at home, you don't have to sit in a doctor's waiting room.

I get up after about twenty minutes of lounging and make it to the shower. Thinking primitively, I believe that hot water on my neck will be healing. But when I emerge, I still need to keep my chin high and my neck unswaying; in this posture I feel regal putting on my shirt and tie. Yes, I am going to work. Doctors never admit to illness. We never admit to illness because 1) it would mean we should go see a doctor who we'd never completely trust (knowing all our own small, secret mistakes), and 2) becoming a patient naturally takes away from our identities as doctors. These two classes of beings, doctors and patients, should not to be mixed in a single person.

Downstairs, my wife has absurd suggestions like, "Why don't you stay home today?" My wife asks if I don't want to take something stronger, but I assure her that a good old nineteenth-century product like aspirin is fine. She calls me an "anti-doctor" and I bend at the knees to kiss her goodbye.

"What do you think it is?" she asks.

"I don't know."

"Probably tension," she says.

"I'm not tense about anything."

"Yeah. Uh-huh."

When I get to the office, Marie asks me what I've done to my neck and she is disappointed when I say I don't know. When she asks me what I think the problem is and again I say I don't know and mumble something about 'spasm,' I can see that she will never refer any friend of hers to me again.

●

I ride up to 9A. The muscles along my neck are stiff as curtain rods. The aspirin is not working.

I go into a supply room to look for a soft collar, one of those wide, tan belts that circle and immobilize your neck and make you look like you've been the subject of a magician's trick gone wrong. I rarely go into supply rooms anymore. They are delicatessens of supplies, walls of wondrously named packages:

>   cotton balls
>   scalpel
>   heat lamp
>   gauze sponge
>   povidone
>   brown jugs
>   sterile sheets
>   arm-board
>   saline bullet
>   urine hat

syringe 1cc-60cc
tape—3-inch
empty evacuated container
ice bag
silver towel holder
kling
rectal therm kit
saline bullet
minidrop set
recipient set
reconstitution set
limb holders
wound drainage bag
cath plug
salem sump
carrington kit
dale binder

I am getting old; half these things I don't have a clue
about; a bum neck and confusion among the tools of my
trade.

I can't find a soft collar. I grab a few tongue depressors
for my kids, some new gauze pads and some tape for our
medicine cabinet at home. I remember a friend of mine in
medical school calling, as a gag, the Association of Tongue
Depressors (we tried to imagine if the building that housed
this organization was tall and skinny) and getting their written materials. Their motto, we learned, was: "To strive for
safe, sturdy sticks."

●

Lynn approaches me.
"I think you've been a good influence on George," she
says.
"Oh yeah?"
"He's been helping out all the older patients he can
find."

"In what way?" I ask.

"He's helping them take strolls down the hall. He takes their arms. He's helping them into chairs for meals. He's feeding them instead of grabbing their food. He's a riot. They love him. He's great with the cranky old babies. He just puts them in their place."

"He's not getting in your way?"

"Of course he's in our way. Some of the girls don't like him, but nurses believe no one can do work as well as they do it. I just get him to help me make some beds if Housekeeping doesn't show up. He doesn't mind. Now that's what I call a cardiac rehab program. He thinks he's leaving soon, so he just wants to help."

I have to try George again with the idea of a stress test. He's giving the world his darting inspection. ·

"Any new thoughts about taking that stress test we talked about?" I ask.

"Educate the fools, you'll find a good many," he says. Every time I speak with him I get a little lost.

"So does that mean yes?"

"I think not," he says. We are in siege. George has a life I'll never really know and a past I can only guess at.

I blurt out, "If you don't take care of this heart condition of yours, you know you could die."

It is an overused device; trying to scare patients into what we think is right for them, a way of creating momentum and adding some mythic dimension to the next decision.

"That wouldn't be a tragedy, now would it?" he asks me.

I'm a little angry at him: if he refuses our help, why did he come to the hospital?

My neck and its wild geometry of pain begin to taunt me again, I have to leave and sit down somewhere, and when I do I think, Who am I stalking here?

•

I walk directly from Mr. Dittus's room to the X-ray department on the third floor. The step onto each stair rattles my neck and makes me wince. I'm not sure why I need an X-ray if I believe that this is all muscle spasm and X-rays only show bones. But I am drawn to the third floor. I want to make absolutely sure that this isn't cancer.

There is a waiting area crowded with stretchers and the transport staff is hanging around in one corner talking about the Patriots and the Celtics until they hear the name of the patient they steered down here called. Then they troop over to the stretcher and push it and its occupant into the small, overchilled room where the X-ray equipment is kept. When I notice one of the X-ray technicians whom I recognize from escorting my own patients down here, I pull him aside.

"Larry, could you take a picture of me?" I ask.

"Of who?"

"Me." I realize that I know his name but he doesn't know mine.

"What kind of film?" he asks me.

"Neck."

"What kind of neck film?"

He means: what are we looking for?

"I have no idea," I say. My brain has shut down. I am the patient not the doctor. This is why it would be useful to have a doctor of my own, to reassure me, to explain that I don't need an X-ray. Of course, if I were an ordinary patient I would have waited to get an appointment with my doctor, I would have been kept waiting in his or her office, I would have waited my turn behind all the stretchers.

"We usually start with a lateral shot," Larry tells me. I think he's smirking.

I wait until one of the rooms is clear. Larry stands me up against the film and gives me sandbags to force my arms to extend downward. He leaves me for a moment, I hear the click, and the returns to relieve me of the sandbags.

"What happened to you?" he asks.

"No idea," I answer.

Out in the anteroom, the film rolls out of the developer and drops into a tray. I stretch to pick it up, the pain finding new spaces along my vertebrae.

"Good luck, man," Larry says. "Why don't you take it over there so one of the docs can read it." He sees that I am helpless.

A kid, a doctor-kid, a small bearded man in training to become a radiologist, grabs the film and asks, "What do you got?"

I don't want to show it to him. I don't know him and he's junior, a novice. I want a senior opinion. But I'm not going to grab it back now that he has his hand on it and is putting it up to the light box. My bones look white and durable. My bones' borders are straight, athletic, and healthy. I know their names. Radiology is like sixth grade history; there is a map called the body and we learn map skills: thirteen colonies/ 206 bones.

I don't want to hear what this little man says. I don't trust him.

"Normal," he says. "You can't see everything with just this one angle, but everything I see is OK." Hedging. But I'm partially relieved. I see no reason to have a senior person read the film: why second-guess this perfectly respectable young man. I have the answer I am looking for.

Still, despite the good news, my neck is locked in a position of nose-up cockiness. Although I have only had this pain for a total of three hours, I am beginning to feel a traveler's sense of fatigue and apprehension.

I take my X-ray (this time by elevator) up to the Rehabilitation Medicine Unit. In the gym, where the real action takes place here, I see leather straps and crutches and sleek prostheses laying about. There are large tumbling mats that I remember from high school, and parallel bars. Floor-to-ceiling mirrors put all the nurses and patients in the right frame of mind; there is sweating and laughter.

I knock on the door of Dr. Fitzhugh, the director of Rehabilitation Medicine. We know each other from the cafeteria as two regular 1:00 PM lunchers. We don't know each other well and when he opens his office door and sees me, he knows that this isn't a social visit. This is reinforced when he catches sight of the X-ray in my hand. I'm sure that he figures I am going to ask him for a little informal advice about a patient of mine, and he invites me into his office. When he closes the door, the walls feel close and the ceiling high; it looks to be, disconcertingly, a perfect cube of an office. Yet the place is so ordered it looks as if Lady Macbeth cleaned it, although it hurts my neck to stare down at his desk.

He is not much older than I am, with gray hair and a sharp nose. He is wearing a blue blazer as he does to lunch. He directs me to a University-emblazoned chair and I see there are no soft options up here in Rehabilitation. If you are badly injured, paralyzed or stroked, there will be no delicacy to your recovery. I begin to feel nervous. Neither of us sits.

"An X-ray," he says, after a short hello.

"Mine," I say.

"What happened to your neck?" he asks, taking the film from me and putting it up in front of his small window that looks out on a concrete wall three yards away. He quickly puts it down.

"I have no idea," I say yet again. "I just can't move it without severe pain in my shoulders and down the spine."

He moves to my side and his fingers move into the pain area without causing too many new sensations.

"The X-ray is fine, you know," he says.

"I'm not much good looking at neck films," I say. "Especially my own."

"You wouldn't see it on a film anyway," he says.

"See what?"

"The facet. Your pain is probably a facet problem."

I feel panic set in. It is amazing how fast I transform into the man I was before becoming a doctor fifteen years ago. I have never even heard of a facet joint in the neck causing such a problem. If a patient like me came to see me as a doctor, I would throw up my hands. I do not ask Fitzhugh how he knows this about my neck; it would be too embarassing. What kind of doctor would he think I am?

"You have some options," he says. "What do you think about manipulation?"

119

"I can't have a chiropracter work at my neck," I tell him. He could break it and that would be that." My friend Patrick and I often discuss becoming PFL, Paralyzed For Life, making lists of all the ways this could happen from sky-diving to body-surfing. Patrick and I share this great terror, Patrick also keeps a cache of other medical horrors in his desk, mostly photographs of horrendous conditions clipped from medical magazines, snapped penises, six-inch-deep wounds, digital gangrene.

"They wouldn't break your neck," he says impatiently. "But if you don't get manipulated this will probably come back at some point. It's not going to get better on its own. The pain is probably from the spasm that is trying to compensate for you being out of line."

This military phrase "out of line" has become a spinal phrase and a character assessment. I figure he's kidding, this MD talking about sending me to a chiropracter. I have never heard of such a thing: MDs refer their patients to MDs.

"Any other choices?" I ask.

"You can take some aspirin and get this roll that you put under your neck when you sleep so that your head is immobile. That way some of the spasm may disappear."

"Where do I get the roll?"

"I think we have one down the hall. Cindy can get it for you. Your neck will probably feel better in a few days." He is edging us both toward the door. "Of course, the pain could come back, seeing as you don't know what caused it." Hedging so I don't blame him.

"So, nothing very serious," I say, hopefully.

He doesn't answer.

"So, not much for me to do but wait," I say.

"That's my quick opinion." He sticks out his hand for me to shake.

That's when I realize he has been uncomfortable talking to me in this informal way. It has been awkward for him: should he ask me to take off my shirt so he can really examine me, or should he accept this incomplete history-taking and poking? What does he owe me, just another of his hospital's doctors, one he doesn't even know very well? Did this count as an office visit and should he start a medical record on me for his files? Was he now my doctor, and if things don't go well, will I call him back, will I sue him? I am just another doctor without a doctor short-cutting the system, placing him at risk for litigation, that's what he's thinking. He wants me gone.

He steps out into the corridor with me and yells for Cindy (the proximity of the gym makes everything informal on this floor), who appears quickly in white sweats and sneakers, a tall blonde with a headband and a remarkable amount of energy.

"Could you get my friend here a neck roll," he says.

I don't catch the name brand and I'm sure I wouldn't have heard of it. I shake his hand again and I hear his door close behind me.

I walk down the hall with Cindy, a hall that is even more cluttered than 9A what with the huge leather balls and the abbreviated sets of four stairs that I imagine a cartoon animal stepping off as a prank. Cindy goes into her office and comes out with a "roll," a firm leather cylinder the length of her forearm and wrapped in plastic.

"You're in luck," Cindy says. "It's my last one. It costs twenty-five dollars."

I gulp at the price. Moments before I had been a doctor who knocked on Cindy's boss' door, had a private, fee-less visit. Now I have to pay up twenty-five dollars. My feeling of entitlement has disappeared entirely. The price is too high for an object I could make at home by tightly twisting a towel.

"If I don't buy it, do you have any other suggestions?" I ask.

"For your neck right? Yeah. You could roll up a towel," Cindy informs me.

I thank her as I walk with her back down the corridor to the elevator. I ride down with a baby strapped into her carriage, and her mother. The youngster is twisting and moving her arms in a swimming motion, trying to escape. I remember my own swimming, how I would have to put this daily exercise on hold until the pain disappears, and then I realize that the day before I had done the crawl for the first time in months, instead of just the breast stroke. And as I try to turn my neck to the side in the crawl's breathing motion, the pain shoots through me again. I smile, because now I can understand the reason for this trouble, then I reach into my pocket for two more aspirin.

•

Who paid for my neck X-ray? No one; certainly not me. If I had had a blue ID card and had had it stamped by the radiology department secretary and sent to Billing, and Billing had charged me for the eleven inches of Polaroid film that my neck fit on and had charged me for the Radiologist holding my X-ray up to his lightbulb and saying, "Normal," I would be out ninety-five dollars. But I don't have a blue ID card.

My X-ray was unofficial. It never happened.

The Haircuts would not sleep well if they knew.

•

Sometimes, I pass a colleague in the hall and we start talking our doctor language. Visitors pass us and can't understand a thing. It's always a surprise to me that everyone doesn't understand our jargon. After ten years of marriage, when my wife uses a word like ventricle (a word she wouldn't have spoken before she met me, although she knew it for a crossword fill-in), she is so proud she stops and flexes a bicep. When I stand with colleagues in front of an EKG monitor, talking about heart block or ectopy or some other great, evocative medical term, as the heart rhythm moves by left to right across the screen like a clown pulling an endless handkerchief out of his sleeve, I feel competent. We talk in tag-phrases because we can't always remember all we need to. We have a tag-phrase reverence. We use words like "noncompliant." We use them so often and so seriously that they spread too quickly and destroy their helpfulness. Then we continue to use them, crudely. Like on my index cards, so I can capture my patients in a word. You can't talk this talk without having some passion for it, if only for its exclusionary value. My wife tells me that when doctors talk doctor-talk we are hard to take. Patients are in a foreign land; we are too.

I walk back to my office listening to the noisy trees, the screeching crows and larks. I have no satisfactory diagnosis for what's wrong with my neck. It is in some way humorous to know how inadequately I have given my history to all who have asked about my neck in the last six hours: my wife, Marie, the X-ray technician, Dr. Fitzhugh. I told them nothing about my swimming; any relation to my pain had not occurred to me. Adding the crawl to my repertoire the night before had not seemed dramatic or worth considering.

I have thought many times about taking a history but less about giving one. Giving a history meant trying to make sense of it, putting it through some kind of rough analysis. It meant placing my pain back into a life filled with activities, into a week of hugs and lurches and rushes and shrugs, all of which might have had some bearing on my neck. Memory is revision, and I had edited out the crawl.

It's cool out, the sky is white and I think of the chiropractor I was advised to see. Thinking of that satyr—half doctor, half wrestler—makes me think of the medical self-help book a patient thrust at me the other day. In it, I read that the causes of disease and pain were criticism, resentment, anger, guilt, jealousy. (It had left out swimming.) The message: The Cure was within us, we already possessed what we sought most fervently from doctors. The same message offered at the end of the *Wizard of Oz*: wizards perish so that we may believe in ourselves. Wasn't there truth to this? Wasn't Dr. Fitzhugh a magician without magic? Facet pain indeed. Who did he think he was? I had exposed a conjuror. My neck still hurts.

I had taken off my beeper when I became a patient so when I get into my office I learn that Peg has been paging me. When I call her back, she answers from Mr. Dittus's room.

"I'm with Mr. Dittus now," she says. "And he has a visitor who I'm sure you would like to meet."

I take two more aspirin and head back up to 9A.

•

I meet Peg by the nurses' station. I tell her that I can't tip my head to look at her as we speak (she comes up to my chest) because of the pain. She ignores my complaining.

"You friend Mr. Dittus is a delight," she says.

"He's probably less strange than he first appears," I answer. I'm already used to Mr. Dittus.

"He seems like a nice man." Peg gives most people the benefit of the doubt. "But not your average honest, hard-working, responsible type," she says.

"But you say he's got a visitor?"

"A friend," she says. "Whatever that means."

"The way he laid out his life, I wouldn't have guessed anyone would be stopping by," I say.

We walk down the hall to Mr. Dittus's room together.

When I get inside the door, Mr. Dittus points at me and says, "Here's the guy who says something on this jigger is way off the mark." When he says "jigger" he lifts the cardiac monitor wires that are clipped to white bullseyes on his chest.

His friend, who is sitting next to him on the bed, stands and extends his hand. His hand is as heavy as a wrench. His eyes are a soggy pale-blue and his nose is shaped like an onion. He is wearing a green duckbill cap.

"Morris," he says, pumping my arm, which sends lots of pain into my neck. "You the boss of this casino?"

"Hello there, Morris," I say. I appreciate his enthusiasm. "Peg and I are trying to come up with a plan for your friend Mr. Dittus and his heart."

"Coca-cola and salt. That's all I need to get well,"

George informs us. Then he stands up and does a little choreography, up-tempo, knees bent. He does some fast side-shuffles and shoulder hitching. He looks preposterous.

"How do you two know each other?" Peg asks, trying to get some control of this scene.

"Cards. We play cards," his friend says. "I had a wife. She had a horror of cards and flies. But she loved picnics, and turkey, and then she died, so now I play cards. "

I am beginning to understand why he and George are friends.

"You've known each other a long time?" Peg asks.

"Maybe six years. I used to play in a big band. Clarinet. Every Thursday at Chan's in Woonsocket. A strange career. Played in front of the bar. What a bar: wide and smooth. I'll never forget it, though I don't go back there anymore."

"George takes pretty good care of himself at home?" Peg asks.

"George was born on a sofa, did he tell you that? His mother was an amputee and she took off her leg and used it for a pillow so she could have him." Morris gives a huge laugh. "Kidding, boss, kidding," he says.

As Morris speaks, I watch Peg. She is always animated and appears to take in a enormous amount of information all at once. Her eyes scan every face trying to bestow warmth, but also checking that all is in order. She never lets a vague expression cross her face; she seems intensely interested. She has to have great patience. But I can see that no matter how benevolent, frustration is not far ahead for her.

"He's an awful card player, as you can guess," George says.

Morris says, "You know, in this country all the bills are the same size, which isn't very practical. In most countries, they're different sizes or colors, blue for a one, red for a five. Throws off my betting living here."

"Do you live near Mr. Dittus? Could you come by and check the pills he's taking every day?" Peg asks Morris, looking for some practical help, but I know it's hopeless and so does she.

"Did he tell you that we always have Mountain Dew and hot peppers when we play poker?" Morris answers.

"How far do you live from each other?" Peg tries again.

"He carries four packs of cards wherever he goes," George says.

"And he's one of the best liars we have," Morris says.

"You think that you will be able to help your friend when he goes home?" Peg asks.

"Live nowhere near him," Morris says. "How is his heart doing anyway?"

"He thinks I brought a heart attack on myself," George answers for me, lifting his chin at me. "But I don't remember feeling particularly bothered by it. And she thinks I should be taking all this more seriously, but I think the danger is in taking it too seriously."

"Always some sorrow without being sad," Morris tells us.

"I wouldn't be sad it I were at home," George says. "When am I going home?"

Peg and I excuse ourselves.

Out in the hall way a pair of old women shuffle by wearing wigs that could never pass for human hair. A sick crow of a man heads for his room.

"Not much help there," Peg says.

"No," I agree, but I am thinking about Morris' line that the hospital is like a casino. I think there is some deep truth there. Of course there are no green game tables, or red carpets, or soft rock emanating from craftily hidden speakers here. The hospital is reinforced concrete; it is inexpressive and functional; there are fewer mirrors. But in the same way as a casino, time disappears. And the hospital is the greatest of all democracies of chance.

"No. But I didn't even think he had any friends," I tell Peg.

"We just need to make clear that proper plans need to be set and that he shouldn't leave until they are."

"*You* tell him that he's staying," I say. "I can't stand telling him anymore."

"He'll take it better from you," she says.

I go back to the room alone. I think: it's like the tension between the governed and the governing, (a tension that also exists in love affairs): who is in control and what resistance will there be? Control is at the heart of most things.

Standing next to his bed, I say to George, "You know there's no cure for heart disease. To take care of yourself, you'll need to take some medicines and you'll need to see a doctor regularly, and we need to think about the best arrangement for that to happen. This is very important. And I know you'll be able to do it, I'm fully confident you'll be able to do it, if you want to."

I am looking at the floor as I speak. I am trying to be upbeat and I have always found extremes of enthusiasm embarassing.

"Sounds good," George says. George has put the full responsibility on me. In some ways, I prefer the state-of-the-art consumer. Ask. Doubt. Question. Be vigilant. Train yourself to understand. George's trust puts me off; I have to think for him and me. Patients should want to know the meaning of their symptoms, but George doesn't.

"We are just planning ahead," I say.

"Usually, I don't even plan ahead enough to buy green bananas," George tells me. Morris waves and I leave again.

•

As a doctor, I'm often asked about the future. Out of my white coat, I'm hardly ever asked, except by my wife who wants to know when I'm next cooking dinner for her. In the hospital, everyone is anticipating. The future naturally seems better to them: they want to know. But they also want guarantees. It's a tall order. If I am the guesser in these instances, they are the second-guessers. What they don't want is pain and abandonment.

Last Sunday, when Scott, our neighbor and fix-it man, went up to clean out our gutters, he found rotten wood along the soffit. As he tore it away, he saw that squirrels had been there. After my dismay over what I would need to pay Scott to fix this stretch along the roof, I realized that squirrels moving into your house was like being sick. You may hear them behind the walls, chewing the wiring, tunneling, you may not. When you find them, you need to get them out.

I really do scare patients, sometimes, with my predictions. I make them worry about what can go wrong. Most of the time though I say, "I don't know." What I give them too often are imprecise and disheartening indictments.

Most of the questions I answer are about the future. If a generalist like me is a specialist in anything, it is in answering questions I can't possibly know the answers to.

When I have a bad day, I think of all the medical jobs worse than the one that I have. I keep a newspaper clipping stuck to my refrigerator with a banana magnet. It's about the interrogation of a terrorist bombing suspect. It reads: "The FBI arranged for a doctor to examine him to determine if he had been tortured. But the FBI declined to reveal the results." A doctor who examines terrorists for the FBI; not my idea of fun.

I think about two things as I drive home. Mostly, I think about putting my neck into a bath. My wife and I call our bathtub "Churchill" because the Prime Minister used to take two baths each day, entering them at ninety-eight degrees and having his valet add hot water until the temperature reached 104 degrees; to me and my wife, it seems that this is the appropriate way to bathe. I also think about my use of the word "cure" with George when I told him that heart disease did not have a "cure."

Cure has an ancient ring to it and makes me think of *The Iliad*, which I read first when I was studying to be a doctor. The mortality rate in *The Iliad* has been calculated at 77.6%, I remember reading, and the thirty-one blows to the head recorded by Homer were all lethal. Trauma was high on the list of Homer's concerns. It was also the first time in history that an author wrote about the war-wounded getting carried off and treated elsewhere (on nearby ships in this case). Medicine has certainly improved since then, but the idea of "cure" hasn't evolved that much. In Homer's book, cures had to do with trauma and blood. Cures were obvious, despite the fact that a true grasp of bleeding came later (with tourniquets, invented soonafter people started shooting guns).

Yet "cure" still doesn't mean anything too exact outside of wounds and skin and bones and surgery; we are still primitives. Sutures are obvious, but disorders that are only inside (like George's heart disease, or my neck pain) are hard to imagine, even with knowledge of anatomy. Suggested cures of what is inside and imagined offer only limited certainty and there is no elation with limited certainty. In *The Iliad*, when your bleeding stopped, you picked up your sword again.

Neck-weary, I can't use my side-view or rear-view mirrors very effectively so I look straight ahead and drive at twenty miles per hour, radio playing, windows open, passing houses with porches, blue mailboxes, a straight mile along a well-known joggers path watching the frenetic dogs gulp fresh air.

•

First thing Thursday morning, Peg pages me.

"I just saw one of the residents who you work with. He tells me that you're planning to send Mr. Dittus home over the next few days. Is that right?" She sounds miffed.

"When we come up with a good plan for him," I say quietly. I had mentioned to my team the idea of getting Mr. Dittus home as soon as possible.

"After what you and I saw yesterday afternoon, I don't think that's going to happen real fast. So I think you should let your team know," Peg lets me know.

"Well, we're going to need to talk about this some more," I say.

What I mean is: I am going to send him home when we think he's medically fit; you do what you can for him in the social work realm before that date.

"Yes, I think we are," she says. "When?" It seems as if she has turned suddenly from an ally to a high-toned challenger. She makes me nervous.

I have heard it on television, but never from a patient of

mine: Doctors shouldn't play God. On television, this attribution usually has to do with the content of a medical decision. Should life-sustaining treatment be given? Should it be withdrawn?

If I do, in fact, sometimes *play God,* I believe it has nothing to do with the content of the decisions I make. If I am like God, it is because I am intimate and impersonal at the same time.

•

I always feel a great fondness for those patients who appreciate me. I enjoy being allowed, yet another day, into their privacies. I wonder if George Dittus appreciates me. In my mind, he is cleaned-up, improved, respectabilized from the George I met three days ago, and he needs me.

I realize that it is a manufactured privacy I get to know about my patients, not the privacy of home, which is wholly different. I never see these patients in their homes making salad. I never see them with their children. I know only certain elements of their gloom. If I passed one of my ward patients a week after discharge as I walked through the local mall, chances are I would not notice them and I might not remember them when they stopped to say, Hello, Look at me, I'm better.

For many doctors the intimate details learned during our short encounters are enough.

It is nearly impossible to explain to other people why I enjoy George, a man who laughs at his own jokes and likes jello.

But as I think about it, I understand that he makes me think of how my father has been described to me—stubborn, independent, unpretentious, mildly uncaring about his own health. They both had red hair.

•

A few years ago, after the birth of my second son when my wife was breast-feeding at 2:00 AM and I couldn't get

130

back to sleep, I went into our den and wrote a letter to my father:

You would be eighty-eight this year. Thank God you're not.

Eighty-eight is too old for anyone. Too many complications, too much sadness unless you're incredibly lucky, and you weren't. At ninety, weight and age moving from opposite directions reach equivalence. I've known only one ninety-year-old without serious slippage. And that itself was a problem; his friends were all dying or dead. You wouldn't have been one of those Arizona, pitch-and-putt retirees, all white chest hair, jackass pants and thatch shoes. You would have hung around the east, taking on the New York freeze. Tough guy, carnivore, Bronx-born schoolteacher, teaching winter a lesson.

Your wife is still here, my mother. Twenty-four years your widow. She hasn't gotten near 88 and her mind is a weakness, although you're still on it. She has few mental means, a failing memory. She has in that brain the young you. Unfortunately, she's not sentimental; she doesn't share. Not that I'm looking only for pleasant stories about you. I'll take the bad with the good. At my age, it's odd that I am asking for stories at all. Sometimes I don't ask; I make the stories up since your wife won't talk about you. I bring her a fiction and ask her if that's the way she remembers it. "Who remembers anymore?" she answers. She only wants to know, often six times a day, who hired the aides hanging around her apartment.

So who can I ask for a sliver from your life? I get tired of running my own memories over and over. I'm looking for someone to trade with me; I'll give you two 1977s for a 1973. Your younger brothers are still alive, sharp, conspiracy-minded, writing editorials to their local papers. To them, you were a hero, a figment, a romance, you were gone from the house first, the smart one, the handsome one, the one with talent. I can't get details. "You want to know about when he was young?" they repeat. "Everyone in our family was born old and sick." They will share pharmaceutical and political advice, not memories. My mother is losing her memory, but they bury theirs. I am a nephew, and nephews aren't worth so much. Last time I saw them, I traded each one an op-ed piece idea for what they remembered of the night Billy Jean King played Bobby Riggs, the night you died.

Every few years I see a man who looks like you. Looks like I imagine you looked. Having you die when I was thirteen frees me to make things up, as I've said. I have no memory that I have to protect, or hold to. I catch a sharp-nosed profile that looks familiar, a wide-shouldered tall fellow with uneven teeth. I see thick red hair. I look closely at all men with red hair. I feel I've met them before. Is that you in there? The funny thing is I didn't even know you when you had red hair. It was white already. But what I hear from your brothers and my mother is red hair. In my mind, this has been transformed to: All people with red hair know something about you; they are your kin. I want to ask for their memories of you. But I stop myself and just stare. I love red hair on men, women, children. I wanted my children to have red hair. My remaining hair bronzes in the summer sun, but I did not have enough chromosomally to overcome my wife's corncrake black and push my boys toward auburn.

There is really no one for me to talk about you with, so I'm glad to get a chance to write, to catch up. I am done dating, which is the second-to-last time in life you get to talk at length about parents, the last being when their bodies and minds start to cause trouble. My neighborhood pals care mostly about their kids' interests—snakes, karate, soccer—their wives' lost voices, new business schemes, the price of slate, their shade flowers. And the parts of their own parents that are attriting, that require attention—uncemented hips, swan-necked fingers. My wife heard all that I had to say about you when we were dating, and my sons are not old enough to ask much. They will get the photos of you, but also photos of me, plus my clothes, stethoscope, library, furniture. Who knows what they'll keep.

By the time I got married, I had lived more than half my life without you. My new bride missed meeting you by fifteen years. By then, I didn't know where you were buried, couldn't describe what your voice sounded like, wouldn't have even mentioned you during the wedding ceremony. Even then, I couldn't remember details about you. I would sit in bed and try to remember everything that happened one day when you were there. I thought that I could sit down and go backward through a day, all we saw and said and did together. And when I failed at that I tried to remember one afternoon with you, or one morning, or one smell, or one texture. And when I failed, sorrow, which I had always assumed would bring insight, simply became sorrowful. These days, when my boys see me still struggling at this task, heart-wounded, they know to comfort me.

Here is one thing I got from you: I love my sons. This is not unusual I suppose, since it is the primary function of fathering. But I love my boys in a way that takes into account your long absence, in a way that perhaps not all fathers would describe: I'm in a rush to love them. I feel the need to squeeze affection into a short space of time. Looking ahead, I am prematurely disappointed that they will grow up. Shameless, pushing, extravagant, I have a love as fast as light. They don't mind me mostly. They say I'm silly, crazy. I love when they come into my bed during thunderstorms. I love clipping their nails. I love the way their writing curls. I love kissing them when they're asleep and don't know I'm there. I love the diameters of their wrists and ankles, the pebbles of their vertebrae. I look forward to reading their camp letters.

It's hopeless trying to recapture details of you. Instead, a new and unusual form of memory has become available to me. I begin to think of those things you had missed doing with me. I begin to think about events in my past that you didn't attend, that took place after you died, and I imagine us at them together. Graduations, birthdays, concerts. I didn't miss these occasions; you missed them. So I give them to you. I imagine activities: the two of us side-by-side pulling on long elastic-ribbed black socks, evening walks to the letter box, helping adjust each others' ties. I simply place you in scenes I did remember, and I made sure you have a good time.

If an adult writes to a parent it's usually seeking reconciliation, or money, or both. If an adult writes *about* a parent, it's usually for revenge. I wish I could say that you ended in madness or guilt or bitterness or pure fury, broken from a dark emotional life. I can't. I wish I could say that you left me with moral clarity, with an unshakeable faith in something, with old-home quotable prescriptions. You didn't.

I last wrote letters when I was a morbid teenager, after you died. By morbid I mean I thought too much about you. When I learned what morbid meant, I became a doctor, although now I know doctors use the word differently. Some days I take care of people with red hair, or widows who have grown sons trying to imagine what's coming next, sons who make things up. I take care of eighty-eight-year-olds until they've had enough. Now and then I take care of men with exploded hearts. Despite the complications, I try to keep them alive.

•

Doctors get from medicine what readers get from novels: some penetration of privacy. For most doctors, it is enough to know the itches, the types of wedding bands, the sounds of breathing. We know, or should know, every bit of our patients' appearances, and how they feel. This is enough.

So when the surgeons I sit with read, they read thrillers, which are thick books of facts (and are not really novels which involve manners and privacies). In some ways, thrillers remind doctors of the hospital: the mystery, the disturbance, another tour of violence, the chase, and finally, a return to equilibrium. Equilibrium is what the best thrillers achieve, and is what doctors hope for as well.

•

At two o'clock, I visit George.

His blood pressure is way out of whack, perhaps higher than I've ever seen in a patient, and it is causing him problems. In the past hour he has had a twinge of the same kind of chest pain that brought him to our emergency room. His blood pressure has to be controlled. I decide to start him on the usual dose of a medicine I don't usually give but which seems to be popular among my students. No one is with us in his room as I stand over him, injecting this medicine into his IV tubing (his nurse is getting us a second vial of the stuff just in case the first does not work).

Suddenly, his blood pressure drops fast, faster than you can imagine. He is headed toward shock, his pulse thready.

George looks glassy-eyed. He is fading. His breathing becomes heavy and slow. I can taste my spit getting saltier, my chest tightening, as I watch him start to go out on me. There is a noise, a buzzing, inside my head.

I scream for the nurses who come running. When I look at the vial, I realize that I have accidentally given ten times the correct dose. As I hand it over, I purposely pinch the tiny tube, cracking it, draining what is left. Fear makes my arms sweat.

We give him fluid intravenously, lots of it, although we know his heart may have difficulty handling the extra load this soon after his heart attack (he has refused to go to an ICU); we have no choice. It is touch and go for a good hour. His blood pressure finally begins to return to an acceptable range.

George's nurse looks at me, and George, dizzy and pale, looks at me, but I am silent. I tell neither of them about the mistake, that he was close to dying because of me. I offer no awareness of what has happened and the empty vial offers no evidence against me. My reputation is strong. If necessary, I could say the dose I gave George just had an unpredictable effect: a lie. I could say that his heart, stiff after its injury, reacted idiosyncratically. I leave the room mumbling about our need to change his medications, go to the Men's room, and vomit.

Almost immediately upon leaving the ward, I come to believe that I have done nothing terribly wrong—George is sick to begin with, which caused his unusual response to the medication I had given. I recognize, by the time I get back to my office in a daze, that I am being self-serving, but also that nothing irreversible has been done.

There is little more I can say to anyone. I am not looking for consolation.

I go home early to play with my children. My wife is surprised to see me at 3:30 on a Thursday afternoon. I am surprisingly patient with them, she observes. They still love me.

After my boys are asleep, and I am in the bathroom with the door closed, I start crying. Sometimes I surprise myself with the tears I'm holding. I am remembering one afternoon near the end of my first year of medical school.

The priest spoke, words agreed upon during years of such occasions, and then the dirt flew. There was no sound of earth on pine; sandy piles rose silently between the small black urns, maybe thirty that stood upright in the unusually shallow university-owned grave. I was dressed like my classmates in dark suit and heavy shoes.

The final amen was mouthed and we scattered soundlessly. We had driven to the cemetary separately and each us headed back to our cars. Overhead, jets mutely descended onto a nearby airfield, their rumbles arriving long after. The ceremony had been strange: a mass-grave funeral for those who had willed their bodies to the medical school; no relatives, no crying, no reminiscences. My participation was involuntary; I'd been chosen at random, like the others, after the Dean had insisted on some student presence.

As I made my way over sunken stones, a small old man slipped from the shade of a monument into my path. He was distracted by private thoughts and moved forward with tiny steps, his knees ahead of his curved body, his hairless white arms in rolled-up shirt sleeves although it was April and still chilly. He was talking to himself.

"Thank you for coming," he said just as I passed him, just loud enough to be heard.

"Are you speaking to me?" I asked.

"Yes. Thank you for coming. It was very kind of you. Very kind indeed. I'm sure my wife would have appreciated it. She was in one of those vessels you just buried."

I didn't know how to answer. There had been thirty cadavers dissected by the gross anatomy class, five students to a body. I started to explain this to the man. "I don't know which one was your wife."

"I'm glad there's a grave," the man continued. "It would be terrible if I had no place to come and sit." He stood wobbling. "You must be a medical student. They mailed me a card saying there would be a ceremony now that you've finished with them. I had hoped I would get a chance to speak with one of you."

I heard him say "finished with them"; I was ready to be castigated, lectured on duty and disgrace.

"So I thought I would come. We had a small service when she died three years ago, but without a burial I never felt quite finished. It's odd, don't you think, that you never saw her alive and I have forgotten what she looked like? I try to picture her, I have photographs of course, but I don't have a good memory anymore. She was born not far from here you know."

I wanted to escape. The old man craved a listener but whatever bond this gave us, it didn't seem reason enough to stay. I started to turn away but I was already back at the silver table, the yellow tarpaulin stretched back, the clean scalpel making bloodless lines on the naked figure. I often worked in the lab in the evening, the one-way windows, tinted outside so no one would look in, became mirrors themselves at night. After two hours of that silence I would return to my apartment, switch on the radio, phone friends. The corpses had green plastic tags on the wrists and ankles, coded in numbers. There were no names attached, no histories, no causes of death. That helped.

"When she died," he was saying, "I was away from home. A nurse was with her."

The man took a step onto a crescent of pavement and waved a hooked finger toward the stone bench with a chiselled design embroidering the rim a few feet away.

"No, but you have no interest in this," he said apologetically. "I don't know why I bother you."

"Your wife, what was her name?" I asked.

The man's empty hands opened and closed. "Ruth. She was a beauty when I met her. 'A spirited girl,' my mother called her."

I wondered if the woman I had worked on was the same wild girl. He told me her story.

As he spoke, I remembered that after one day with the body at close range, there was nothing mystical left. I felt like astronomers must have after studying the universe without locating heaven.

"It is good though that she gave herself to you students. Studying the parts helps you remember, doesn't it? To you there must be nothing to death. You will see it all your life. You have chosen to see it," he finished.

"Yes. That's right," I said, as he rose, and still talking aloud to himself, headed off.

As I drove home I realized: for a few moments I was a conduit for his love.

Through the door I hear one of my boys snore. I rinse my face with water. Those who live simply and can depend on me as their doctor have a secret of living I admire and envy. It makes me sad that they can never know the whole truth about me.

•

PART THREE

THIS MORNING, WHEN I called Gresser, I was glad that I hadn't mulled it over long. It was Friday, the end of a bad week, I wanted to see Gresser, and that was that. I had just finished looking through the autopsy report.

What were my expectations when I called? I half-expected him to be sinister. I was sure that once he heard my father's name he would at least be defensive, and if he was an alarmist, he would hang up quickly. I knew that I would have to hide my anger toward him. Quarrels, accusations, would have cut short any hope of conversation.

The fact is I know nothing about my father's final hours. I know that he was sick, had been for years, but not how or why he died. He was fifty when I was born; the night he died I was two months short of my fourteenth birthday. I was a boy. I had no chance of understanding.

The Call:

"Is this Dr. Marcus Gresser?"

"Yes it is."

"My name is Peter Cave. Some years ago you took care of my father Samuel."

"Yes I did." Without a moment's pause. "That must have been twenty-five years ago."

"Yes it was."

"You must be in your thirties."

"I am."

He was asking me questions. So calm. Like he was expecting my call.

"What can I do for you?"

"I was wondering if I could come in to see you. To talk about my father."

"You know I'm retired now."

"I didn't."

"I closed my office five or so years ago. It got to be too much."

"My father had heart disease."

"Yes he did, I believe."

"I have the autopsy report."

"If you need some help understanding it, I'd to glad to . . . ."

"I'm actually a doctor now, but I had a few questions."

"A doctor. I see. Let's go over it then."

"I was wondering if I could come down to see you."

"Where do you live?"

"About three hours away. North."

"Yes, I suppose that could be arranged. Let's see. I don't remember too much about your father's case."

"It's been a long time."

"Yes it has. I'll need to go into storage and pull out his chart."

"I appreciate it. Can I come down today? It's a good day for me."

"It's worth coming if you want to go over things I suppose."

"It's been a long time."

"How's your mother?"

"She's well."

"Haven't seen her in years. She still live around here?"

"Yes she does."

"What time will you get here?"

Our conversation was over fast. He was businesslike and trusting. I wondered how my father had come to use him. They were in the same social circles. Word-of-mouth probably. Fate.

I have no idea what I am going to be able to say to him but I have things to say. Whatever happens at the visit I figure I'll be better off.

When I told my wife that I was going to see Gresser this afternoon, she put her hand on my shoulder and said, "It's the right time to go."

That's when I got a dizzy feeling and was glad she was holding me, steadying me. I knew the sudden weakness was just my grieving taking over.

I am leaving in two hours.

I am to meet Peg on 9A before I go.

I take my time getting to 9A, stopping to see a few patients on other floors. I pass the monotonous handwriting of the EKGs on the screens at the nurses' stations. I see lunch being served on the lower floors, prematurely, but who really cares about time here. The food has almost no odor, food without garlic or lemon or wine or oregano, overboiled vegetables, almost farcically tasteless chicken. I pass many rooms where I have seen death, but the dead that I remember are gone. I remember the rooms, and in some cases the particulars of their occupants. Yet the dead are simply and quickly replaced by the next near-dead.

I stop in to see another of my patients who has cancer and has been here for three weeks. An elegant wasted old man, his relatives are visiting and he looks bored. When I come in, his wife grows panicky and I immediately begin planning my escape; I only wanted to say hello. From rooms where my patients are mingled with the patients of other doctors, I hear yells. Like the screams of a hunt. I hurry past. At the end of the corridor on 7B are that ward's demented tied to chairs, two men sticking their hands into imaginary holsters, drawing and shooting the passersby. I look into cool rooms with calm light made for the blue skin of the sick.

I think of the conversation I had with Peg earlier in the day. Peg, tiny and pudgy as ever, talking to a nurse, twisting her neck as if she were a corkscrew rising with its job done. My own neck was only slowly improving.

"Mr. Dittus tells me that he is ready to go home, but I don't think he is," she said.

"Well, he may be later today if he continues to move around without any problems, without having any more chest pain," I answered.

"I don't think that he'll be ready even then," she said.

"Because?"

"Because he's had two heart attacks in two weeks and he still doesn't have a clue what happened. Because he didn't take any of his medications at home before, and we're just planning to send him out with medications again and he won't take them. If he dies, we will feel pretty bad," she said. "We've been over this."

I did not want him to die and did not expect him to die. I wanted George to live. He couldn't live in here—not George. He was a funny, hustling scavenger. I wanted him to escape, with me as an accomplice.

"I agree we'll feel awful if something bad happens, but it's possible that nothing bad will happen," I said calmly. "And if he wants to go, he's going to leave, and we can't stop him."

I felt protective of George and I knew that he would do well at home.

Somewhere deep in me I also knew he might not do well. The heart isolates itself from all that it knows sometimes.

"Do you think he's competent to make the decision to leave?"

I saw where Peg was leading me. By 'competent' she meant: Does George Dittus have sufficient decision-making ability to participate in the decision about his discharge? Should we listen to what he wants? *Competent* seems like such a bland word to rate something as important as a person's thinking.

What Peg was asking was: Is George truly able to understand the relevant information we give him, is he able to appreciate his situation and its consequences, and communicate to us what his problems are, why he needs to take his pills? In other words, is he able to explain to us why he makes the decisions he makes at all? If he cannot, we could keep him against his will until we are satisfied that he will be safe at home.

Nothing is worse than keeping someone against their will. To my mind, it is like killing.

I try to think of this competence business from the patient's viewpoint. If I were a patient, and I made what seemed to be a bad treatment choice, I would want my doctor to really try to figure out if this choice was simply a bad but competent one, based on deep-seated goals and values

146

possibly more important than my health, or rather, an incompetent one, that is, I could not even understand the choice I was making. If it turned out that I had made only a bad choice ("bad" here means, most often, one the doctor disagreed with), then the doctor should try to talk me out of it, but failing to do so, should give in to my wishes. If, on the other hand, my doctor found me to be incompetent, I would want him to protect me from the potentially harmful consequences of an impaired decision.

Both Peg and I wanted George to be in charge, but what Peg wanted most of all, when she asked me, "Do you think he's competent to make the decision to leave?" was for George (whom she claimed was packed and ready to go) to make sense of his choice to us.

With the patients I like, *I don't care* if they can make sense of their predicament; I have a tendency to let them do as they wish.

I told her, "I don't know if he's competent or not, strictly speaking, but he makes a lot of sense to me and I don't want to keep him here against his will. And I think he's probably competent."

"And I don't want to send him home to die of another heart attack, and I think he's probably not competent." Peg told me.

For me, nothing spoils work faster than endless debate. I wanted a decision, the motion of going ahead. I didn't want to keep George hanging. Peg and I had come to different conclusions, probably not far apart on a "not-able-to-make-a-decision" to "fully-able-to-make-a-decision" scale, but far enough.

"So what should we do?" I asked.

"Get another vote," Peg said.

We decided to call a psychiatrist in to interview George and act as a tie-breaker.

"Who's gonna tell George that he will be meeting with a psychiatrist, me or you?" I asked.

"I'll do it," she said, and the anger that I'd been feeling toward Peg for stirring up all this trouble sunk a little bit. "A

147

psychiatrist is coming to see you," still has a bad ring to it for some patients.

Why was I angry at Peg? To say that I felt betrayed by her would be overstating it. But I felt bad a little. I knew that she was just doing her job. She was just offering her opinion, which I asked for in the first place. But the thought of a psychiatrist evaluating George had me worried.

I realized that I had taken a sort of pride in George. In a week, I had grown accustomed to his quirks and could interpret them for other people. When I told my wife that George was one of the most eccentric patients I had ever seen, I was being boastful. I was taking credit for him. The more eccentric he became the more I respected him. He was like one of those relatives we all have who we're fond of despite their bad disposition, who are annoying to most people we know, but whom we find funny nonetheless. George ordered white cake with white frosting at every meal; didn't that demonstrate a form of self-knowledge? Still he was not an attentive man. I did not believe he really saw what was happening to him or around him.

I was angry at Peg because while a psychiatrist could easily find that George is incompetent and should not be sent home—which would mean that I would be judged cavalier in my approach to his care, that I would be putting him at risk if I were to send him home—I think of it the other way around: I am protecting George from us, from the dangers of The White Life.

While I think of most patients as transients who visit me for a short time on their way to discharge (domestic or celestial), I think of George as a true transient, one whose constant movement predated his admission. I think of George as someone in a permanent state of departure. Holding George against his will would drive him crazy; he'd be furious. I do not want George in a rage. Trying to convince an angry George that his care as a captive is in his best interest would be hard work and heartbreaking.

On my way to meet Peg I get a call from a nurse on 9B telling me that Mr. Elderkin has died. He woke for breakfast, ate an English muffin and went back to sleep. They found him in his bed. It is the first death I have had since my mistake. This news gives me a gloomy presentiment of another certain failure: I will not get George out of the hospital and home. It drives me back down into the sadness I thought I had escaped.

I stand and look out my office window over the parking lot, the cars in lines like graves. Sleeping people never die in their own dreams; this is conventional wisdom. They slip away from the robber who pursues them; they sidestep the knife blade; they avoid getting crushed. So when people die in their sleep, it's nothing they ever imagined. The dream has ended, they must think. Not that I can really imagine any of this, for Mr. Elderkin or anyone else.

I keep repeating an expression my grandmother used to use, "Dead to the world till morning."

I am paged: I am already late for Peg and she hates tardiness. When I call the number on my beeper, the voice says, "Doctor, it doesn't matter to me what you do. When I'm ready, I'll go home."

It is George. I know what he's talking about immediately. "How was your visit with the psychiatrist?" I ask. I am surprised that Dr. Marsh has gotten to see him so quickly. Peg had only called him an hour before.

"Doctor," George says. "Between you and me, he is a very touchy guy. He asked about my parents and I said to him, 'I'm not telling you. Go dig it out of the ground.'"

"You didn't like him, huh?" I feel secretly pleased. I am competitive with my colleagues in this way.

"You're all crooks," George says. "But this one looked puzzled a lot."

"Like when?" I ask, trying to get a feel for the interview.

"Like when I told him I hated banks and salesmen. He acted as if he found out something shocking beyond belief. As if anyone liked them. I bet he's the sort of guy who's not gonna let it die down either. And after all the wonderful conversation we shared."

"Probably not," I say.

"Your social worker friend said she was coming back too."

"I'll stop by late this afternoon," I say.

"Don't knock yourself out," George says.

I decide to call Dr. Marsh. I try him twenty times and when he picks up, I can picture him with his standard bow tie, his red ears, one soft loafer dangling over the other.

"I don't think Mr. Dittus is equipped to care for himself very well at home," Marsh informs me.

Although I don't know him well, I think that Phil Marsh sees himself as living and breathing his patients' lives after only one interview with them, but underneath he has a cold, mean eye. He never gets jovial until after work, I imagine.

"He has strange habits, I know," I say.

"The man dries his wet laundry in his toaster oven," Marsh says.

"I didn't hear that one," I respond.

George is bizarre, no denying it. I know him, but I still don't know much about him at all: how he thinks of death, who his ghosts are. The house he grew up in, what was it like? I try to fill in the lives while I am watching and touching and listening, (as you would in any romance) but I haven't been altogether successful with George.

"He wouldn't tell me much," Marsh says. "He's very determined to get home, though. Very determined. He had fifty reasons why he had to leave in the next twenty-four hours. But I think his disease is a mystery to him. He believes that it has to do with eating too much white cake."

Narration, wanting to tell the story of sickness, comes so easily to patients that it is always a surprise to find someone who won't tell their story. This sort of person is particularly bothersome to psychiatrists who depend on the tale. "Tell me about that," psychiatrists say. But with George I had the feeling that telling was his undoing and he knew this about himself.

"He knows more than he lets on," I say, defending George.

"He's obstinate, you know? He's almost too determined

to leave before things are settled. I'd say he's obsessed with getting out of here."

Or he sees what's coming, I think to myself. According to Phil Marsh, George's determination has become a psychic disorder. I am beginning to think we've picked a lousy consultant and I will be obliged to ignore his suggestions.

"I tried to figure out what it feels like to be George Dittus, and I couldn't do it," Marsh tells me.

"What did you tell him?" I ask.

"About what?"

"About going home."

The game of medicine is played with the cards under the table. I know this.

"I told him that it would be you who would have to decide when it was medically safe for him to leave."

Now that was the right thing to say. So I risk the next question.

"But do you think he's competent to decide when he's going to leave?"

"Probably not."

What comes to mind first is: more fuel for Peg. I think of her small face, like a cat's, boneless, and therefore impossible to interpret. Then I think: Marsh has blown it here. He's simply wrong.

"Does Peg know your opinion?" I ask him.

"She was there for my interview with him," Marsh says.

All the doctors I know have two recurrent fantasies. The first is to be their own boss. The second is to stump a panel of experts. To take what had once been your own patient's perplexing symptoms, a diagnostic dilemma that you have already solved artfully, returning the patient to health, and bring this patient's history and examination findings before a panel of know-it-alls for their opinion. To bring them a case that will not leave them amused, while you know the answer. There is no doctor who doesn't dream of this. Watching the experts spin and doubt themselves. Watching them sweat and in the end, guess wrong. And to give them your diagnosis and hear them say: "I was conned," "Oh, it couldn't be that. "

I feel this sensation of triumph-to-come when I hang up with Marsh. I believe that George is competent; he'll do fine.

This is the first time in a day that I have a clear conscience making a clinical decision. I have been walking around fearful of making mistakes. Drawn out fear becomes doubt. Again I am a man with considerable authority. I feel it. Today, you can't take liberties with me.

"So I hear that Marsh doesn't consider George competent," I say to Peg when I finally meet up with her on 9A. I am feeling strong.

"I think he felt it was a close call," she says, and I can almost hear her gloating. Or so I imagine. Peg dominates people with generosity.

"Did you tell George?"

"I'm not sure what to tell him."

"Well, if still refuses to have a stress test, but he's doing OK, I still think he should go home. I mean, what are we going to do with him?"

"We need a plan," she answers. "Especially since he's not really competent."

"I think Marsh is wrong," I tell her.

"I know you do," she says. "But he's your consultant. You called him in."

"I'm going to ignore his opinion," I tell her. "Which means I need your help even more."

When doctors are imperious (as I am being), we don't want to be tagged imperious so we make an effort to charm.

"We still need a plan for Mr. Dittus."

"Yes we do," I agree.

"He has no relatives," she says, thinking aloud. "We've met his friend, and there's no help coming from him. If we send Mr. Dittus out, he'll come right back, possibly dead. He can't stay here; he's uninsured." I think of the Haircuts losing money every day on George. "Which means he could go to some sheltered environment until . . . "

"A nursing home?" I say.

"He'd be safe there."

"George in a nursing home? Oh, he'll love that. *You* will tell him that news."

"We may have no choice," she says.

"Now that would kill him," I say. I want to quote her that Hank Williams line: "Lord, I'd have to get better before I could die."

"The reason to send him would be that we could be sure he'd get his pills for the short time that he would be at greatest risk," Peg says.

"That's a little extreme, caging him in a nursing home so he can take pills." I reconsider Julian Barnes' view—pills and bureaucracy; maybe he's right after all.

"I don't think so," Peg says. Which means: you're the doctor and can send him whenever you want, but if you send him now you won't get much of an opinion or much help from me again in the near future, and besides, you're a doctor and should believe in the power of the pills you're prescribing, and the pills won't work if they are not being swallowed so let's figure out a way to get him to swallow them reliably.

I feel that Peg is treating George's coronary disease too respectfully. I have always thought that Peg is curious and well-informed. But here we needed inventiveness. The best doctors think themselves and their patients out of difficult situations. George's situation is novel: what you want is for patients to go home, but many don't or can't, so you stop trying. George *could* go home and we weren't going to let him.

"I think George will be OK at home," I say again to Peg. "We'll explain things again, he will take enough of his pills, and I'll see him again in my office within a week."

"Here's a plan," Peg says, ignoring me. "If he can show us that he can take his pills, we send him home. If he can't, we need a new plan. Let's put him to the test."

As small as she is, she keeps coming up with things that are big and unanswerable.

Then I realize the strange reversal that's taken place: a doctor wanting to send a patient home under perhaps suboptimal conditions and a social worker taking the high road, forcing pills.

Peg is the opposite sex. Opposite is an unfortunate word, but telling.

I pause at the 9A lounge to stare out at the tugboat. After I hung up with Gresser this morning, I went back into my study and picked up my father's autopsy report which sat in my desk drawer. It was six pages long and stained brown with age. It was divided into two parts, External Examination, which took up only a paragraph, and Internal Examination.

"This is the body of a well-developed, well nourished white male appearing the stated age of 64 years, measuring 176 cm. and weighing approximately 230 pounds. Examination of the head reveals purple mottling on the face. The pupils are dilated, equal and round. The chest is unremarkable. The abdomen is moderately distended. There are two old surgical scars, right and left paramedian, measuring 25 cm right and 23 cm left. The genitalia and pubic hair are normal for a male. The extremities show pitting edema."

This is the way doctors describe the dead.

My father.

I am glad that I refused to visit him.

"Death is the side of life turned away from us," Rilke wrote.

This is how my father's heart is described:

"Weighs 600 grams. The epicardial surfaces are smooth and shining. The left and right atria and their appendages do not show significant pathology. The right ventricle measures 0.8 cm in maximum thickness. The trabeculae carnae and papillary muscles are slightly hypertrophied. The endocardial surfaces show whitish streaks. The left ventricle measures 1.8 cm in maximum thickness. The trabeculae carnae and papillary muscles are hypertrophied. The endocardial surfaces are smooth and shining."

When I first read this passage, the phrase "smooth and shining" momentarily gave me a bright outlook; a lakefront, a baby's face, I thought. But it was a mirage of comfort. The phrase describes my father's heart, lifted from his dead body, in the light, aloft, in the hands of strangers in some hospital basement twenty years ago.

I stop in to see George before I leave for Gresser's. Twenty-four hours ago I nearly killed him. He tells me that he's not had any more chest pains since his arrival in the hospital.

"You know I stay to myself," he tells me. "I hardly ever go out to people's houses. They talk and talk; people are either bores or windbags. And most of what they say is lies anyway. And anything you say, they tell other people. Stay at home and you don't get in trouble, that's my motto.

"When my mother died, I took down all the curtains. I never put anything else up, but upstairs is in the trees and no one can look in. My mother's house was built to last. That's not true anymore, as I'm sure you know. They are built to wear out. That's the way people want it. I wouldn't sell it. Not for any price. Got my yard, got my bird visitors, burn my own garbage. You own your house, you do as you please. Cats. I have ten. Yard cats. I let them get food on their own. That's why they're fat."

He is sure of his destination.

I think of George, roaming this hall, scavenging from other peoples' trays like his cats.

His room contains defiance in the form of a packed bag, even if it is only a small, blue, plastic hospital bag with a drawstring. His lunch has been served early.

"If this is coffee, please bring me some tea. But if this is tea, please bring me some coffee," George says.

"What did you order?" I ask.

"Oh, never mind," George answers.

I decide to tell him straight out. "Listen. For you to be able to go home safely, you need to show us that you can take your pills. Your pills are going to keep you alive and you need to take them." I feel as if I am overdoing it, but I go on. "There's no one at home to help you take your pills, you have to do it yourself, and you've already told us that you haven't been taking them since the last time you were here."

"You're all crooks," he says, biting into his grilled cheese sandwich. "You want me to stay so you can collect some more money. I know you're paid for every day that you come and see me. And you send some of your other doctor friends to see me, so they can get paid too. I know the routine."

I ignore this. "I've simplified your schedule of pills so that you only have to take them three times a day." I know how difficult it is for most people to remember once a day; I can't do it. "You are scheduled at breakfast, lunch and before bed. You've had your pills delivered to you in bed since you've been here, but it won't be like that at home. So here's your new job. All you have to do is remember to go up to the nursing station to get your pills with each meal. If you don't miss any doses the rest of the day, home you go." This was the plan that Peg had come up with and I had agreed to. I want to add: and *I'm rooting for you*. But I don't.

"And if I don't take my pills, then what, Herr Doctor?"

I was afraid of this. "Then we'll need to make other plans."

"Code words, code words."

I am amazed and moved by George wanting the details. I expect him to be hesitant and uneasy. I feel the power of the threat I hold; I did not expect to have to threaten him. "It means you might have to go to some facility where you could be watched everyday."

"Like someplace other than a hospital."

"Yes."

"Like someplace like, say, what?"

"A place like a nursing home," I say.

"A nursing home. A place like a nursing home."

"Whatever you decide to call a place where you don't miss any pills until you've recovered from your heart attack."

"I have recovered from my heart attack," he tells me.

"Almost," I tell him.

After five days with George I know that he never asks for favors from anyone. Nothing shocks him. He draws conclusions but will explain none of his thinking. He arches one eyebrow and looks at me with pity; I am still trying to solve a problem that isn't a problem.

If he'd been a different sort he would have argued. He would have threatened or cried or swung at me. Still, I am surprised when all he says is, "I see."

I open the button on my white coat. I remember David saying: A white coat is to a doctor what a balcony is to a dictator.

"Let's start now," I say.

After he puts down his jello-loaded spoon, the two of us walk out into the hall and go to the nurses' station together. "Go ahead," I prod him.

"Pill time," he says to the only nurse standing there. She knows the plan; I had explained it all to her on the way down to see George. She hands him a thimble-sized white dixie cup with one oblong blue pill and one yellow square and he downs them, no water.

We shake hands. A contract.

Our hospital is not a prison but we are using it as one. George will simply be waiting for me to release him. I will come and go while he stays. I will be back this evening after seeing Gresser.

"Swamps," he says. "Swamps fascinate me," he says. "Highest concentration of life. Opposite of a hospital." Then he heads back to his room.

Giving this news to George makes me think of when I sang "Rock-A-Bye Baby" to my infant son. I used my sweetest, cooingest voice, but the lyrics were treacherous:

> When the bough breaks the cradle will fall
> And down will come baby, cradle and all.

•

I like to go to work every weekday, and it feels both wrong and unpleasant to be driving south. I want to be at my hospital as I am every Friday afternoon, preparing my patients for a quiet weekend. I did not turn the care of my patients over to anyone as I do when I go away for a week.

As I drive, I remember the house I grew up in with my father: blue living room wall-to-wall carpet, not enough bathrooms, screened porch in the back like a cage, yellow refrigerator. In the thirteen years we'd been together he'd given me his values: a belief in calm, sensible behavior.

There was nothing tragic about his death. He was sixty-four and was very sick with heart disease.

The drive is familiar. Route 95 south through Connecticut—this old factory town, the mirrored insurance buildings—the northern suburbs, boats docked in little coves. What frame of mind is appropriate for this visit? I feel a deep unease but also an exhilaration. As with every visit to a doctor that I've never been to before, I forget all my questions. Somewhere around Stamford my mind goes wildly, nervously blank. I am convinced that if my father had lived into my college years I would never have become a doctor. He distrusted doctors, considered them pretentious, greedy, heartless—or so my mother said—and as I thought of Gresser it was in my father's terms. My father was right: doctoring is a game, an exalted game. Oddly, I recall very few other things my father actually said to me. Within a year of his death I remember that I couldn't hear the sound of his voice anymore.

I cross the Tappan Zee and drive down the Palisades. It is a beautiful morning. The road is empty and there are deep green woods on my right side, a mowed emerald meridian to my left. I can see the Hudson River to my left as well, the cliffs of northern Manhattan. Whatever Gresser tells me won't be accurate. It's too messy.

When I return to the hospital this evening, if someone asks me where I've been all day, what will I say? To the doctor? To New Jersey? I rushed to an appointment that I was twenty years late for? It was a little crazy, but also the truth and unchallengeable and serious.

Around Greenwich, I am filled with the most specific hate that I have felt in years. Not the disgust that I feel toward the house inspectors who missed my termites, or the porch repair guy who overcharged me, but real hate. I want to avoid the depressing and the false and the wistful with Gresser, so perhaps I should just come out and tell him I know he killed my father. But he's dealt with irate family members before and he would do what I would do, wait me out, let me control myself, pretend to be generous and admit nothing of the complex and horrifying truth.

I am confused. I want to see who he is, but I'm afraid it will be a waste of time. That there will be nothing to say.

After I have driven for over two hours, I am dreamy, not paying attention to the shiny morning.

Ahead, to the right in the woods, there is a scampering, and coming out of the woods (driving seventy miles per hour this happens very fast) a red and black blur shoots out toward my lane. As I get closer, I see that the animal has wings and just before I hit it, it lifts over my front hood, barely clearing my fender and I see its underside and pedalling feet. It is a turkey, a wild turkey. Landing on the green meridian I watch it rush away toward some high grass. A pretty good leap for a bird that doesn't fly.

A wild bird. In New Jersey?

Last year, a week after her husband died, a friend of our family's called one morning to tell us that there was a fly in her kitchen who she thought was her husband. It was him; he was back; she was sure of it. She watched the fly, and it watched her, and then flew off. While I am not desperate enough to believe that this wild bird on the highway is my father, I must admit that the idea occurrs to me. I think of my father as I see the bird again in my rear view—his double chin and sharp knuckles and sunburned forehead—but then I have been thinking of him the entire trip.

I keep an eye on my mirror as the road curves to the left and the bird seems to have disappeared, but I know he is there.

When Gresser answers his front door I think: to understand is to forgive; even the first steps to understanding are
impermissible. I hold myself back.

When I shake his hand, I feel that I am giving something
up.

He is a thin man, nearly bald. His glasses, delicate silver wire frames around wide lenses, make his head look
small. He has pale lips, a trace of a white mustache, and an
O of a mouth like the tip of a rifle. He leans on a cane and
wears a white shirt open at the neck, gray pants.

"How was your drive?" he asks.

"Fast," I say. I am tense and unyielding.

"Why don't we come back to my office. Having my
medical office in my house was one of my best decisions,"
he says.

I follow him down a narrow hallway toward the rear of
his house, a doctor and his patient. My father had taken this
walk. Gresser's medical office is a simple room with a low
ceiling in the rear of the house. Looking over his large oak
desk, which claims the center of the room, there is a picture
window. His backyard is a walled garden that appears well-
tended. There is a rhododendron in bloom, six feet tall,
planted before I was born. An ornate, colored glass lamp
sits on a table in the corner and an oil painting of a marketplace hangs from one wall. His desk is empty except for a
thick medical chart in its manila folder and a fist-sized
model of a human heart. The heart has blue arteries on its
surface where they should be red; it is all wrong and sim-
ple-minded.

He sits behind the desk and I sit across from him, as a
patient would.

"How old are you now, Peter?" he asks.

"Thirty-five."

"Beginning of your career."

"I've been teaching for years already."

"You look young."

"The first gray hairs have arrived."

"Your father," he begins. His voice is sure and peaceful.

160

"Your father came to me the year after his first heart attack. He was thinking of having a baby with your mother. He was an older man, around fifty I believe, although I wouldn't call that old now." He laughs quietly. The bird feeder over his shoulder has traffic; a chipmunk on the ground picks up the seed-litter. "They wanted to have a baby and your father wanted to know how long he was going to live. He wanted to know if he was going to see his child grow up. He said if he wasn't going to have any input, they would forget the whole idea. A bachelor until age forty-nine, a new heart attack, a new marriage. He had things on his mind. Well, he always had things on his mind, your father. He was a very smart man. No pushing him around. You must have strong memories of him."

"I was thirteen when he died." I am irritated that he keeps asking me things. His excruciating calm is making me grind my teeth in rage. But in moments of stress I almost automatically become poised and self-possessed, which I attribute to my medical training.

"Your father was the sarcastic sort, lots of ammunition to him," Gresser continues. "Knowing him, he probably made a joke out of his question to me although I don't remember his words exactly. Remember, this was 1960 when the typical number of years of life after an MI were pretty few in most cases. Nothing like what you guys can do now with patients. Amazing how much it's changed. Your father knew the score. I think when he walked in, he was against the idea of having a child and your mother was for it. As a rule, I'm careful with people's hopes. But he kept after me, 'Give me an idea,' he asked. I remember that I gave him my advice but wouldn't quote him any numbers and he was angry. He wanted facts, and he wanted to do things his way. So he stormed out of here. He came back of course. Anyway, that baby was you."

I can't sense anything hidden or unseen in Gresser. He is not trying to keep a secret. He isn't going to apologize for anything. He'd had his life, his travel, his dinners out. I could tell that he believed in the simple and sacred parts of medicine, the acts but not necessarily the results. He'd traded heroism for a smoothing over of any rough spots on his conscience. He does not think of medicine as either risky or self-indulgent as I do.

"So what can I do for you?" he asks.

"I have in my head that you killed my father," I say.

"And where have you gotten this idea from?" he asks calmly.

"From the autopsy report. The small section in the beginning that refers to his presentation at the hospital. He had simple congestive heart failure. It should have been treatable."

"He had a bad heart. Worse than you know. He was quite far gone, nearly past the point of help, when he got to the emergency room."

It's what I would have said. I know I am looking for answers he can't, or won't, provide.

Gresser picks up the model heart out of habit or nervousness and holds it, and I know he would have explained its functions in generalities if I had not been a doctor myself, and if he had begun his standard delivery I would have had no reason not to believe him.

"You didn't clear his lungs."

"We couldn't."

"You didn't," I repeat, trying to convince myself.

"What kind of doctor are you?" he asks.

"An internist," I tell him.

"Then you know about the heart."

He'd been with my father that last year and was still loyal to him, I could see. He was the last person to see my father alive.

"You read through the autopsy report," he says.

"Yes I did."

"Well you could see how sick he was then."

I realize that when you spend you life in pursuit of something, particularly something very hard to find like the reason for what happened, it is easy to be disappointed. And that's when I realize that, in a way, this is as close to my father as I would ever get at this stage in my life and I was glad I had come. I can feel my fury settling. All I've got now is Gresser and I watch him carefully. I lean back and link my fingers behind my head, press my palms to my ears as if he were screaming.

"You know he refused to take the medicines I suggested," Gresser says quietly.

"I didn't know. Why was that?" I am confused; the whole visit has been confusing.

"He was a tough guy. He knew best. He wanted things his way."

I feel tired, defeated.

"I think your father would have been happy that you became a doctor. Most fathers are."

"I'm not so sure," I say.

"You enjoy your work? So many doctors today don't." Gresser's career was full of certainty and purpose. He practiced at a time when doctors kept to themselves, believed in good deeds, never credited irony, and were incapable of contrition.

"Usually," I answer so as not to disappoint him.

We talk for a few more minutes. He tells me ordinary stories about his practice, how he had years "full of wonder." He tells me about his sons who decided not to become doctors, and, unflinching, he offers a few more memories of my father.

"What else can I help you with?" he finally asks.

"I'm not sure."

"How's your mother's health?"

"Just fine."

"Will you stay for coffee?"

"I have to get home," I answer.

The whole visit lasts twenty minutes. He shuts his front door before I even pull away from the curb.

It's been a long day. I feel like the Scottish paleontologist Robert Brown who began his daily search for fossils in formal dress and top hat and by the end of the day was nude but still searching.

I smell the sweat on myself, the "fierce goat" under my arm.

I think of George. What I'm doing with him bothers me, nags at me. We have not given him our best, classic care, our diagnostic tests and invasive ameliorations. My daily conversations with him have become banal.

And I have taken one large decision away from him: he can't go home without my blessing.

I get home at 6:30 PM. Before I can tell my wife about my trip she says, "You got a call from Lynn on 9A ten minutes ago."

"What about?"

"She wants you to call her."

"Okay."

"So how was he?"

"Who?"

"Gresser."

"He's respectable. He keeps up appearances."

"That's it?"

"I don't know what to say."

"How about: he's a hypocrite, he's a drunk, he's a fuck-up, he's an unmitigated asshole."

"None of that."

"Okay. Let's move on," she says. "And how were you?"

I cannot tell her that I left Gresser feeling disoriented, disconnected, terribly exposed, though I did; that I was trying not to hit him or run away the whole time I was with him; that I was sad but also close to panic. But she knows. She knows me.

"I listened mostly," I say finally.

"Did you confront him? Tell him what you think, real or imagined?"

"I don't know what I think."

"Yes you do." She is exasperated. She has heard the family myth for years.

"I told him that I thought not enough was done. But what would I have wanted done? Maybe nothing more could have been done. I don't know." The pressure to have immediate feelings exhausts me. "You know my father

164

went to him when he wanted advice about having a child. My father didn't want a baby, but he wanted to know from Gresser how long he had to live so he could have ammunition against my mother's plan to have one. And you know what Gresser told him?"

My wife is a kind woman. Though irreverent, she listens carefully whether or not I give her much. Whether or not I'm trying hard to explain myself, her eyes do not break contact. "What?" she asks.

"He advised my father, 'Your heart is beating. You can't know how things turn out. What's left in life surprises everyone.'"

•

I leave my wife in the kitchen and phone the hospital from my study.

"Morris would like to see you," Lynn says.

"He's back?"

"Yes he is, and he's asking for you."

"Now?"

"He says it's important."

"Now?"

"Oh, give the guy a break," Lynn says.

The service that we provide is not like others'. Our consumers are different; they arrive with complaints before they've paid for a thing, and what we doctors have to offer does not depend on the attractiveness of packaging or price. It does not depend on advertising or even our friendliness. The demands of the sick are always there. The family and friends of the sick call us. They just call.

I kiss my wife hello and goodbye, avoid my kids who would whine for me to stay, and get back to 9A. I will never get home.

Morris offers me his hand, but I avoid it; I'm afraid of its power.

"George is unhappy, doctor," Morris tells me.

"I understand," I say.

"No, you don't. He's unhappy with you."

"With me?"

"He thinks you're not involved enough. He thinks you keep your distance. You don't pay enough attention. This is not my opinion. This is his opinion. He thinks you don't make the greatest decisions."

I look at him with no real wish for honesty. I am stunned. I have this flash to a time when I was a boy and I tried to help a man up off the sidewalk where he was lying and he pulled me down on top of him and tried to squeeze the wind out of me. He had a nasty laugh.

"George won't tell you this, but I will. He's worried you're going to send him to a nursing home. He's worried you will lock him up. I try to tell him you won't, you're a nice man, but he doesn't believe me. You know something's always gone wrong for George all his life. You can't put George in a nursing home. He would die. You would be *killing him.* He would die if you took him away from his collections."

I want to shout: what do you expect? But I'm afraid I'll hear, "Not much. A minimum. Very little."

It has taken me years to learn the extent of my power.

"I'm trying to get him back to his apartment," I say to Morris.

"And to his collections. He collects everything, you know. Paper clips, gourds, you know, squashes, buttons, rope, dresser drawers, whistles, sofa cushions. He hunts down bargains. Just in case."

"Just in case of what?"

"Just in case, in case something else goes wrong, he has supplies."

"He likes bargains," I repeat. I'm curious.

"Things out of dumpsters."

I can imagine George in his apartment crunching around his living room, tiptoeing around precious junk.

"He likes his things and his home," Morris continues. "He's ashamed to tell you he can't go to a nursing home. He says it will make him into an old man. He doesn't even like old people. Everyone likes old people, right? George spits at them. No respect."

"I can't make him go anywhere he doesn't want to go. You tell George that," I say.

"That's good. Because he won't go. He'll die if he goes. That's what he says, and he tells me only half of everything."

"He won't die if he goes," I say. Morris just looks at me.

I go through my day telling patients that they can't live the way that they want to live. I am constantly stealing things they have lived with all their lives: cigarettes, fatty foods. My mind is filled with data, their minds are filled with fantasies and pleadings.

I've always assumed that life is changed by events like heart attacks, but it probably isn't for most people. I want George to go home.

I think about what Morris has said. I do not think of myself as a doctor who distances himself, but perhaps I am self-deluding. George may not even have wanted me to know how he felt about me, but now I know and I am angry and thankful. I am always learning things patients don't want me to know. I wonder how I could act differently. I will try to be warmer, to be friendlier, but I'm not sure how to do it at this point in my life.

The way patients see me is always complicated. I need to make George understand that I care, that's what Morris is saying. But perhaps there is nothing I can do. I try to read the crack on my ceiling like tea leaves, looking for clues. I want George to do well. But there's a lot I just can't say to him. The central truth about doctoring may be that you go through all the motions of friendships with patients without making friends. The crucial moments that doctors and patients share pass, as they never pass for friends.

Occasionally, patients make you see your choices. They force you to make decisions as they do.

In the hall I ask Lynn how Mr. Dittus did with our pill-taking plan.

"He didn't do very well," she tells me. "Let me put it another way," she says. "He screwed up royally."

"How's that?" I ask.

"Well, he didn't come back to get his pills at all. We gave him an hour grace period from the time he was supposed to show up asking for them before we went and delivered them."

"What did he say when you arrived with his pills, when you told him he'd forgotten?"

"I'll tell you what he said to me. He said, 'My father told me 'Some people are put on this earth to be bad examples.' That's what he said to me."

I walk into his room.

"Hey, doc," he says.

"How are you feeling, George?"

"I'm not happy," he tells me. It's very difficult to persuade anyone that they're happy when they're in the hospital.

"No, I suppose not," I say.

"My rent's due. Who's gonna get my checks and pay my rent and my telephone, that's what I want to know?"

"I'll call the telephone company and tell them that you're in the hospital with a serious heart condition," I tell him. I write letters to insurance companies, to employers, to the State Health Department. I can certainly call AT&T for George.

"Have you ever talked to someone at the phone company? They just want to be paid. They don't want to hear your excuses."

"They'll probably understand," I say.

"No they won't," he says, matter-of-factly.

"Well, we still can't send you home. We've got to come up with some plan so you can take your pills."

He screams, "You guys know a hell of a lot about nothing. I'm not a robot. You can't treat me like I'm a robot."

I feel bad for George, and I know, suddenly, that I have to keep trying with him. Even though he's making me look a little foolish thinking I'll be able to send him home. It makes no sense to give up and go to a judge with our case, saying George is incompetent, send him to a nursing home. Because he doesn't want to take a stress test or any other test, and hasn't taken his pills at home? George has probably never tried this hard in his life. The thought of George locked up, a captive in our hospital, disgusts me.

Then I get mad again at Peg. How could she think that George is incompetent? How incompetent could he be with his telephone bills and his car and his apartment? The man has been functioning in the world for nearly sixty years. He makes the mistake of getting admitted to the hospital and meeting her and now we're thinking about committing him. And all the drinkers who come into the emergency room drunk, who spend a few hours drying out, who we know are going back out into the world as dangers to themselves and others, do we think of sending them to nursing homes? No. Peg wants him to be perfectly safe, but who's safe?

With George, Peg and I have become two opposing factions in our own mini Social Protection Agency.

"I know you're not a robot." I tell him. "What can we do to help you with these pills. Why couldn't you go get those pills?"

"I was distracted." He looks toward the door checking to see if anyone is nearby, listening.

"Tell me about yourself," he says suddenly, quietly. "I want to know you better."

I don't feel like getting into it. I'm not sure what he wants from me.

"What I want to know is how *you* are," I say sympathetically, reversing the flow.

"Living, thank you."

It would seem an odd reply anywhere but where I work.

I notice it first in his face, a change in attitude.

"You know, life doesn't stop so easily," he tells me. He seems peaceful, almost happy, saying this.

"I know what happened between you and me yesterday," George continues. "The facts of life."

"I'm fine," he says. He looks at me, full of interest. "I worry about *you*."

The feelings are hot in my face. George sees me for what I am—a man who made a serious mistake. I thought that George was not watching, but now I know he is, and has been.

I call Peg at home to tell her the news that George has failed, but she already knows it.

"George must be depressed," she suggests to me.

"Didn't seem so," I tell her.

"He has to be," she says.

I give her a little bit of her own jargon. "Peg," I say, "depression is about loss, and George feels he's lost nothing. Not even his health."

How do I know this? Because a doctor's job involves a recognition of losses.

"What do we do now?" she asks.

"To make him happy, you need to get over to his house, bring his mail and bank book here and let him write a check for his phone bill and his rent. That's what he's worried about."

Social workers actually do stuff like this: go to people's homes, let themselves in, and bring back needed supplies. While most visitors would snoop, Social Workers never snoop more than necessary. I always ask them to check the medicine cabinet though; I never know what pills my patients are actually taking.

"George doesn't have a bank book or a check book. He doesn't even have a bank account or a checking account, he's told me."

"Go on," I say, waiting for the rest.

"He keeps all his money in cash, under his mattress."

I'm sure there's a long story why George keeps his money under a mattress, but I can tell you that there is no explanation. The unforseeable ways that people live are constantly exposed to me. How to avoid the conventions of past perceptions, that is another challenge for me. Under the mattress? That has to be a joke. But it's not.

I go over to the 9A nurses station to review George's medications and make some simplifying changes.

170

Nobody likes pills. Even changing what we call them has not helped us swallow them: tablets, capsules, caplets, gelcaps. I believe elixirs are taken better than pills simply because the name is magical, but I have no proof of this. Also, a good part of the time, patients feel fine to begin with, so why take pills?

But I have to admit that patients who don't take them are upsetting for me. Yes, there is the simple concern for the patient's well-being. But also, I believe that noncompliance signals a basic lack of fear. And if the patient does not fear their condition, then my authority has been rattled.

What is it that I do to George's pill regimen? I make sure that he only has to remember to take pills twice per day, once in the morning, once in the evening near dinner.

I'm ready to send him home and he's ready to go. I want him to get his pills right. After his failures here, I want him to make a comeback. That's the American way.

I need to go home, to crawl in next to my wife.

People are strong. I've learned this, although I see it as a disadvantage to doctors. They're strong because it's hard to change the body much. It would be hard to make George's coronary blockage go away for long; it's hard to get cancer to reverse its course. Motivation helps. As does the hope of rejuvenation.

A nurse comes up to me and asks me to see some other patients. There are so many. They keep coming, the physically marred, the exhausted, the fluid-spillers, the fabulously weird. I marvel at them. None of them want to be here; no one is here who doesn't have to be. I see a fifty-five-year-old with a blood clot in his thigh who makes wine in his basement. I see an eighty-eight-year-old whose first memory is of having diptheria and being forced to drink peroxide as a cure.

I am allowed to touch them, to examine them for a brief moment (as if we're in love). It is the early part of the night. There's a cozy exposure, like we're in the back of a small convertible. We are allies against a particular future. I smell them. A just-removed moccasin stagnation, a warm, humidified stink.

Thomas Mann was right: "All interest in disease and death is only another expression of interest in life."

They all want meaningful moments with me. But what if I don't? Must I, anywhere and anytime, wring out meaning? Their secrets become, simply, data once discovered. I know that I should not disappoint them or be disagreeable. A great white space would open between us. I feel the dull exhaustion caused by the repetitive duties of The White Life.

But I am thinking about George again. I have thought of him so much this last week. I am still considering his options. I pass patients standing in their doorways like aspiring stars and starlets waiting to be discovered. I pass rooms filled with music and prayer. I hear patients asking in their various languages: What did I do with my life? I pass pyramids of fruit, hearts of candy, all the frivolities finally assented to. I see relatives trying to prevent him, her, from fading away. I see the sharp faces of pain trying to experience full happiness despite the ravishing. I have felt their skin, thin as the skin of warm milk on the back of a wooden spoon. I have felt their necks and shoulders and wigs. I have handled the slippery beads of their bones. I have had them tell me their memories, slowly out of privacy and guardedness. Memory works like an IV set, drip-feeding. I have heard weary courtesies and have offered forced scraps of a middle-aged man's wisdom.

In every room, always, the TV is on. The TV with its continuous run of doctor-shows, the writers afraid of all that I see everyday, afraid of their own relatives really dying. Afraid of the chronic conditions that last longer than a half-hour. The TV hospital seems arbitrary and frantic; sickness is treated like any other chase scene. If I were a patient, I would turn it off. But they don't.

Flaubert: "The public wants works which flatter its illusions."

Despite the fact that I associate silence with loneliness and loneliness with hospitals, I realize that I have never heard the hospital entirely silent, never felt the great size of silence around me. I think of white when I think of silence and loneliness, the absence of color and sound and people. Miracles are white in my imagination. Yet I have never felt a miracle happen in the hospital. I have never seen an angel here or known the force of holiness. Angels and miracles are drawn to silence. My work is all too human, filled with human noises, and some days I wish this weren't so. I remember that line of Annie Dillard's: "The ring of the silence you hear in your skull when you're little and notice you're living, the ring which resumes later in life when you're sick." That's what I hear, that ring.   Last night, my wife and I watched a show on public television that filmed, over several months, a support group of women who had metastatic breast cancer. Although I was reading, I was catching some out of the corner of my eye. About half way through the hour-long show, when one of the women died, I started crying. My wife turned to me and seemed to understand my reaction; she was teary too. She took my hand. It's always surprising that sorrow can run up on you that suddenly though. She thought that I was crying over the women on TV and myself and my father and my upcoming visit to New Jersey.

It was the second time that day I had cried. That's when I told her that I was crying over a man I almost killed.

I have never cried in front of my patients. I believe that crying would seem like a verdict when I should be opposing fate. They wouldn't want me to cry.

That is, I've felt *the need* to cry around some of my patients. But I have not actually cried. It's like those times when you're better off pretending deafness than giving a response. I avert my glance when my eyes fill, as if the situation were a question of modesty. By the time that I get home, by the time I think about the patient who made me saddest that day, I usually feel less shaken.

But there I was crying in my own bed, the book I was reading open on my chest, my glasses slipping and slippery.

I keep trying to find an answer to why I did it and it keeps sending me back to why I wanted to be a doctor. I wanted to be a doctor so that I wouldn't make any mistakes in life. Doctors don't make mistakes. Perhaps I had a fear of being only a man.

As I drove north an hour ago I thought the matter was no more complicated than this: perhaps Gresser had killed no one; my father had simply died. We can probe for oversights, test for errors, but in the end, most often all we can do is unyoke ourselves from the full weight of sadness.

A month ago, I sent home an eighty-nine-year-old woman who was admitted to my ward service after falling at home. She had lived alone in the same small apartment for fifty years. She was not seriously injured (she had bruised her knee and her cheek) and was ready to return home with no real explanation for her fall when she told my medical student that she had fallen because she had been trying to "run away." Run away from who? The six men who had come to rape her in the middle of the night. How had they gotten in? Had this happened before? Why hadn't she told us earlier? And then it turned out that she never actually saw them, that she only heard their voices. They had never actually touched her, but they wanted to. They came every few weeks and had been doing so for years. When we understood that her visitors were fantastic, we asked a psychiatrist to see her. This man wanted to keep her in the hospital; he wanted her transferred to the psychiatric service.

She wanted to go home.

She would be all right, she said.

The psychiatrist insisted that she stay, much as Marsh did with George.

I sent her home. I asked the Visiting Nurses of our town to visit her the next day and the next, and thereafter for a few months. She did fine at home. Her fantasy probably continued although she never mentioned it to me or anyone else again.

I want George out. I want him gone. If I free George and give him his life back, I may feel, for a moment, the old satisfaction.

When my wife saw me crying last night, she said to me in her gentle, forceful voice, "I don't know who you feel more sorry for: yourself, George Dittus, your father or Gresser. You'll see that you're not Gresser. You're not George Dittus because you've never been a patient; you don't even know how to put on a hospital gown. And you're not your father. You're gonna be with me and the boys forever."

I return to George's room. He has just taken a shower and with his hair painted to his skull, he is unblinking, shiny, white.

"You're back. That's dedication," George says. "And I'm really very boring to talk to for you, isn't that right? I always give the same answers. They don't change if they're the truth." George always seems to be looking over my head when he talks, looking into the distance.

"I don't mind," I tell him.

"How's my heart doing?" George asks me.

"I've seen worse," I tell him.

"You've seen worse?" George seems surprised.

I feel a wild helplessness come over me. I remember him saying to me, when I informed him about his heart attack, "It does no good to worry." The destinies of patients and doctors are profoundly and irreversibly intertwined. This is often inconvenient and unfair and we can do nothing about it.

He is sitting in his mustard chair, feet up on his bed, reading a newpaper. He's wearing shoes, black lace-ups. He looks wary.

He is whiter than he usually is, the ugly white of the lipstick teenage girls use.

"I'm still sitting around here," he says.

"We got the pill thing straightened out, don't we," I say slowly.

His eyes get concerned, interested but distant. He is appraising me. He gets up and starts pacing. His fingers are flexing, his eyes narrow. I am momentarily concerned for my safety. George comes to a halt and we look at each other.

I know he blames me. For keeping him too long. And probably for other things. He was ready to leave when we first met.

He seems to understand what I'm saying, and what I'm not saying. "You bet," he answers.

Although we don't have the pill thing straight. Not even close.

I'm letting him leave. I have to. He has a life to lead and what's left in life surprises everyone. He may make all the right medical decisions from here on in. But I doubt it. All that I know is that I have been careful not to judge him too quickly or harshly; I hope he has judged me in the same way.

George's disappearance is my loss. His vividness is gone. But I don't feel bad about this loss. He'll probably be back.

When I finally get home my lovely wife is awake. She says I seem better, but I'm not so sure. I don't have much to tell her.

I suppose you grow close to some patients because you recognize yourself or people you love in them. But when this happens, you want them to leave. You can't stand them any longer.

Mixed results from noble plans. That's what I expect from the next fifteen patients who get transported onto my ward. In the meantime, with summer coming on, I'm repainting my house white.